THE Reignite WORKBOOK

From Burned Out to *On Fire!*

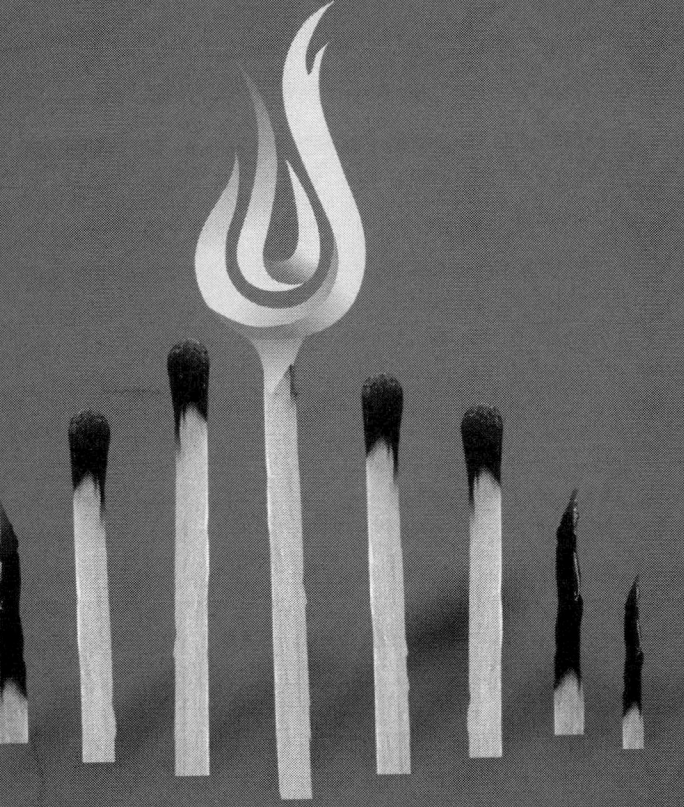

CLARK GAITHER, MD

THE Reignite WORKBOOK

From Burned Out to *On Fire!*

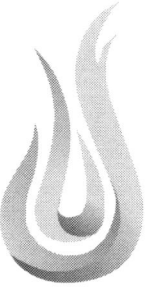

DR. BURNOUT
REIGNITING WITH PASSION AND PURPOSE!

A. Clark Gaither, MD

This *Reignite* Workbook belongs to:

NAME

DATE

"Your future isn't something that just happens to you. It gets decided every day with every decision you make."

All rights reserved.

© 2016 Anthony Clark Gaither, MD
No part of this book may be reproduced or transmitted in any form or any means, electronic or mechanical, including photocopying, recording, or by any information storage or retrieval system, without permission in writing from the publisher.

Copyright Notice

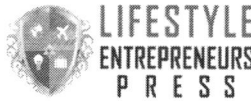

Publisher: Jesse Krieger
Write to Jesse@JesseKrieger.com if you are interested in publishing through Lifestyle Entrepreneurs Press or foreign rights acquisitions of our catalogue books. Learn More: www.JesseKrieger.com

Any unauthorized use, sharing, reproduction or distribution of these materials by any means, electronic, mechanical or otherwise is strictly prohibited. No portion of these materials may be reproduced in any manner whatsoever without the express written consent of the publisher.

Interior layout design by Filipe Dinis (www.creativebuzz.pt)

Legal Notice

While all attempts have been made to verify information provided in this publication, neither the author nor the publisher assumes any responsibility for the errors, omissions or contradictory interpretation of the subject matter herein. The purchaser or reader of this publication assumes responsibility for the use of these materials and information.
Any perceived slights of specific people or organizations are unintentional.

Table of Contents

Introduction

How to Use This Workbook

Why are physicians and other healthcare providers burning out?

My Personal Story of Burnout

Setting the Stage: A Bit of the History of Medicine

Defining Happiness in the Practice of Medicine

    The Public's Perception of the Good Doctor

Defining Burnout

    The Industry Standard Definition — The MBI

    Burnout in Women

Burnout in Men

Stress Versus Burnout

The Causes of Job-Related Burnout (JRB)

The Signs and Symptoms of Burnout

The Scope of Physician Burnout

Is It Our Profession's Fault?

Assessing Burnout: The Maslach Burnout Inventory (MBI)

What Is the State Opposite of Burnout?

The REIGNITE Framework

    Taking the Necessary Steps to Alleviate Burnout

    Review

    Envision

    Introspection

    Your Mental Realm

    Your Emotional Realm

    Your Physical Realm

    Your Spiritual Realm

    Generate

    Neutralize

    Implement

    Transformation

    Engagement

Closing Thoughts

Products and Services

Bio

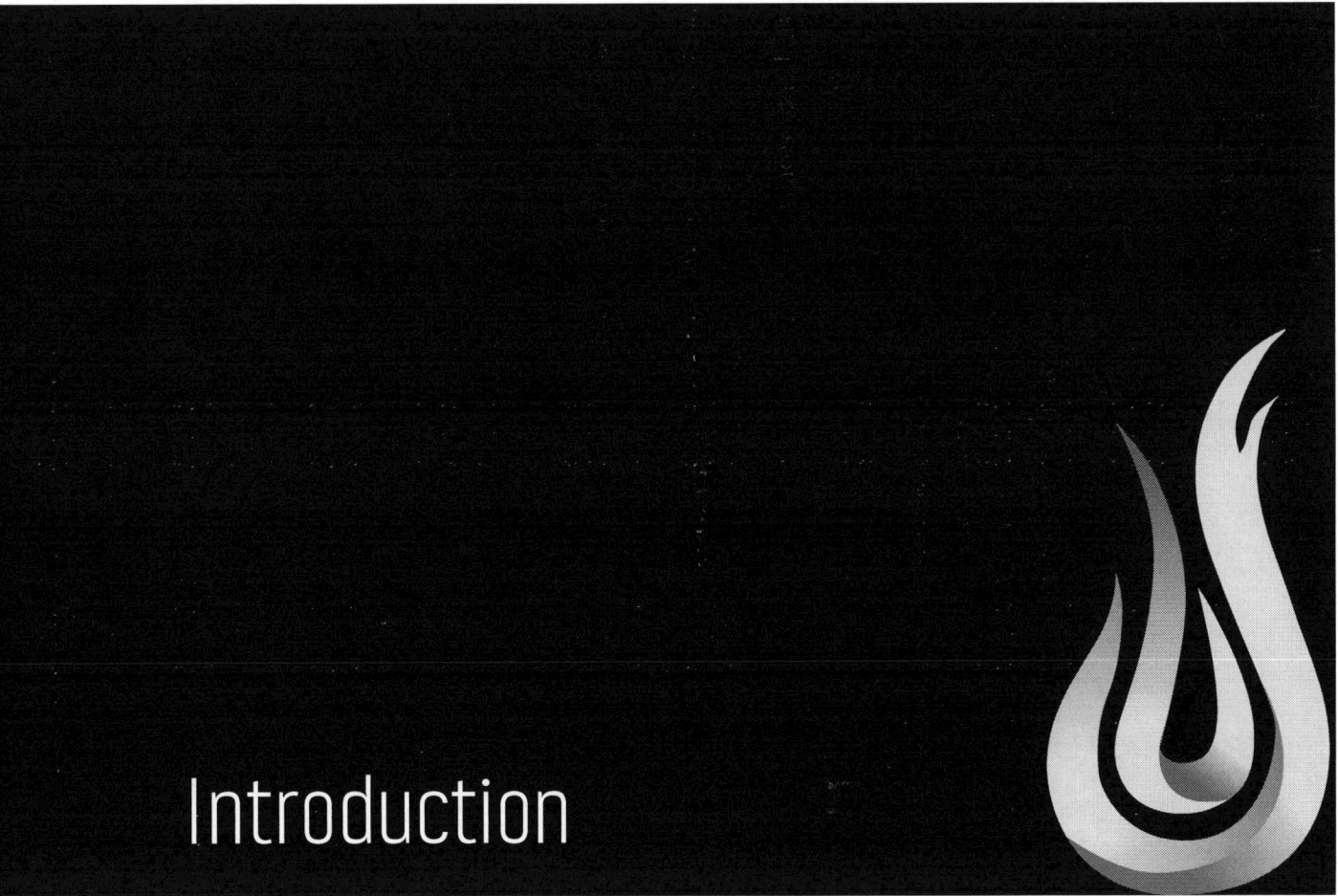

Introduction

The house of medicine is literally on fire, and the doctors are the ones burning. Physician burnout is epidemic among the various disciplines in medicine. To varying degrees, every age bracket and every other demographic you might mention are represented. All of the various medical specialties and subspecialties are involved and none of the data is good.

The result of this is that physicians are reporting high levels of job dissatisfaction. Many are leaving medicine altogether, or contemplating leaving earlier than they might have, due to feeling burned out. Many others are turning to drugs, alcohol or acting out in other ways as a means of coping with on-the-job stress as a result of burnout.

It just doesn't have to be this way.

Whether you are just beginning your career in medicine, beginning to burn out, or are already feeling burned out, this course will help you. This guide contains real-life practical information to help prevent or restore damaged lives and careers due to burnout.

Is it possible to retain or recapture your personal joy and pleasure in the everyday practice of medicine? The answer is yes! The first step of this journey begins on the very next page.

But first I want you to read and answer the following questions. They will give you advanced insight as you move through this course. Print this page out, write your answers in the space provided and date it before moving on.

How many years have you been in practice? _____

How many years did you plan to practice or at what age had you planned to retire when you first started? _____

Has that number changed over time? Circle: YES or NO

If YES, the number has changed, at what age do you now plan to retire or how many more years do you plan on practicing? _____

If you had it to do all over again, would you have chosen medicine as a career or something else?

Circle one: Medicine or Something Else

Today's Date: _____

How to Use This Workbook

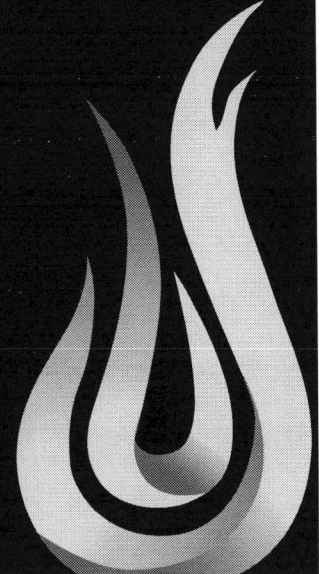

You have been provided the PDF file of this workbook, which contains hyperlinks for accessing additional resource information.

While there is great utility and convenience in opening and reading the source material presented herein from a laptop, tablet or pc, there are some parts of this workbook that request your written response.

Some of the requests may seem repetitious, but asking for similar information in different ways will serve to illuminate central themes in the difficulties you are experiencing. This will create focus and clarity and allow you to better concentrate your efforts for needed change.

> *"Focus magnifies purpose.*
> *Clarity amplifies passion."*

Also, you may wish to make notes from time to time as you proceed through the material. Your notes and responses to questions will serve as a useful list of actionable items.

While on your way to REIGNITE, a red marker will serve as your torch. Use a red marker for answering questions, noting action items and for commitment declarations. Items in red will remind you where you have been and where you are headed — signposts on your journey forward.

For the reasons given, print out a copy of this workbook so you can easily complete and record any requested tasks and use them as a reference later.

In lieu of printing out this entire document you can just print the following pages on which responses are requested:

Why are physicians and other healthcare providers burning out?

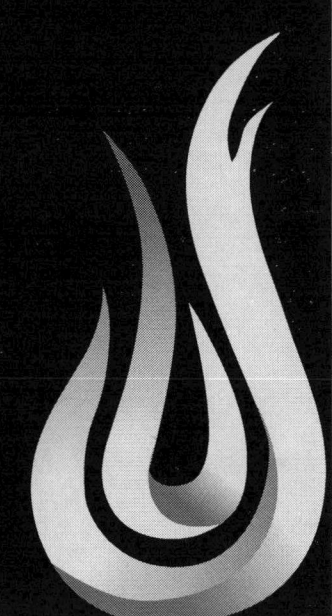

You don't need me to tell you how tough it is out there. Suffice it to say, I do know just how tough it is out there in the trenches of the everyday practice of medicine. I'll share my story of burnout with you in the next section.

I am a family physician. I have been in the clinical, private practice of medicine since 1992. In just that short time period, changes in the practice of medicine have been sweeping and rapid. Every aspect of medicine seems to be in a continuous state of flux. Not all of the changes have been positive.

Here is a list I have compiled of some of the negative aspects of practicing medicine today. I see all of these as interferences in the doctor-patient relationship. Feel free to strike through any you might disagree with and add any that have become a sore spot for you.

The REIGNITE Workbook

- Ever increasing patient care mandates.
- Unreasonable care guidelines.
- Onerous recertification requirements.
- Malpractice worries and concerns.
- Continuous rule changes from government agencies and insurers.
- Falling reimbursement.
- Rapidly increasing costs.
- Loss of autonomy when making treatment decisions on behalf of patients.
- Time constraints on patient encounters.
- CMS/OSHA/CLIA.
- EHRs
- Meaningful Use.
- Pay for Performance. Payer Contacting.
- Managing an increasing number of morbidities among a rapidly growing and aging patient population.
- Managing a practice.
- Employee problems.
- Unreasonable patient expectations.

Can you identify with any of these? Add your own items here:

_____
_____
_____
_____
_____

My Personal Story of Burnout

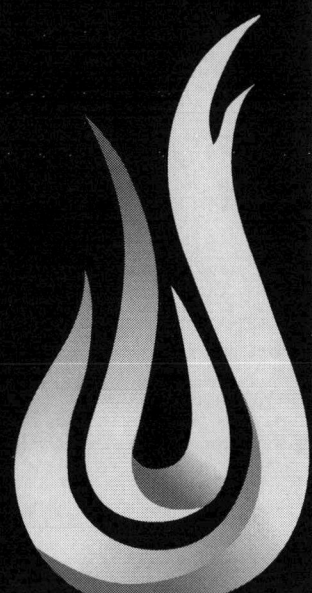

At one time, many years ago, my life had become completely unmanageable. I became an alcoholic, put my career in jeopardy and was ruinously close to losing everything for which I had worked so hard.

I was able to get sober and have been continuously sober since January 23, 1990, my sobriety date. Little did I realize this was just the beginning of my transformation. There was much more in the way of personal disappointment and turmoil on the horizon. Though, I was unable to see it at the time and I was wholly unprepared for it when it arrived.

All of the years I have spent in the practice of medicine have not been great years. Medicine has been good to me and I believe I am good at the practice of medicine. Yet, I have always felt as though something was missing. Have you ever felt this way?

I enjoyed my work when I first began my career. I was very

thankful for having such a great job. Still, I had never felt as though the profession fit me just right or that I fit medicine just right. Does this sound familiar?

The best way I can explain what this feels like to me is by way of an example. As you know, what we do day-in and day-out requires the use of a lot of exam gloves. Over the years I have tried on countless myriad gloves in various sizes from an array of manufacturers composed of various materials — latex, PVC, nitrile, synthetic rubber, etc. I have tried them all.

To date, none of them have ever felt as though they fit my hands just right, not perfectly. I wear them and I can always get the job done while wearing them. But, this "not quite right feeling" is emblematic of how I have felt in the practice of medicine for the past twenty-seven years.

I have never been able to shake that feeling. In spite of feeling this way, I put my head down and worked hard for many years. I was able to accomplish a lot and succeed in many areas of medicine as a clinician, speaker, volunteer and teacher.

I was even fortunate enough to be named Family Physician of the Year in 2002 by the North Carolina Academy of Family Physicians. All the while feeling like I was meant for some other purpose.

This feeling spilled over into my practice. Although it took many years, I developed a dissatisfaction with my job. I came to feel emotionally drained most all of the time. I seemed to be irritated by everything and everyone.

I couldn't wait to get off work and lived for the weekends. At the same time, I dreaded going back into the office on Monday mornings.

Ever increasing patient care mandates, unreasonable care guidelines, rule changes from government agencies and insurers, rapidly increasing costs, malpractice concerns, loss of autonomy when making decisions on behalf of my patients, time constraints during patient encounters, having to manage an increasing number of morbidities among a rapidly growing and aging patient population, unreasonable and burdensome continuing medical education requirements — all of these things contributed to my unrest. Can you identify with any of these?

I felt used up. I was becoming very cynical. I was irritable and unhappy. I felt put upon by everyone and everything. I hadn't felt any joy or pleasure in my work for a very long time. It was only my seventeenth year in private practice and I was a long way from retirement but I knew something had to change.

In 2009 I went to my practice partner and shared with him that I either had to make some changes or I was going to have to quit practicing medicine. I told him exactly how I felt, overworked, dissatisfied and unappreciated. I didn't feel I was making any difference in the lives of my patients. I didn't blame him but I secretly resented him in a way because he didn't seem to feel any of what I was feeling. He, his life, seemed happy and balanced.

The truth is, I had over extended myself in trying to be the "everything to everybody" doctor. I was trying to do too much for everyone around me and not enough for myself. I was a people pleaser and I definitely had a hard time saying no to anyone. Can you identify with this?

I had been reading on the subject of physician burnout and was convinced I aptly fit the definition, well, just like a hand fits a glove. So, I put an action plan together for myself and began taking some steps to fix what was broken.

The first thing I did was go to three days a week in the office. I made those days each an hour longer but I was now off four days out of seven. I took a cut in salary, but I would have worked for free just to feel better and to have a shot at happiness in my work. I began to use the extra time to get my mental, emotional, physical and spiritual house in order.

I resigned from over half a dozen boards, staying on only one for which I was most passionate to serve. I read, traveled, ran and rekindled old interests outside of medicine for which I had previously made no time.

I began to study job-related burnout in depth, its warning signs, symptoms, consequences and treatment. I began to give talks on the subject, and they were well received. I found many colleagues who identified precisely with the way I was feeling.

These steps made all of the difference. I began to enjoy the practice of medicine again. I developed a new patience for my patients. Energy returned. I felt more at peace. I became hopeful for the future again. I began to achieve a more balanced life.

Still, I had not quite put all of the pieces together. That feeling that I wasn't doing what I was called to do never completely went away. It took a few more years in private practice, a convergence of circumstances, and another personal crisis for me to realize that for true happiness and fulfillment I would have to completely transform my life, first by defining and then by pursuing my true passions and purpose.

This has brought me to the present. I have begun to share my experience, strength and hope with others who feel as I once felt — burned out. I have begun coaching others on their journey from silent suffering to wellness.

My transformation has been nothing short of miraculous. I would earnestly hope the same for you. I want you to come to know what I know. If you are suffering from the symptoms of burnout, it just doesn't have to be that way.

Not only does every human being have the ability to change, I believe everyone has the ability to completely TRANSFORM their life using their own unique natural talents and abilities. Everyone has the capacity to transform, to undergo a metamorphosis of the mind, body and spirit in order to dream, design and construct their own preferred future.

- If you feel that you are merely existing rather than living, laboring at a job that you detest where your true passions can not be expressed or where your talents can not be developed or constructively explored, just know it doesn't have to be that way.
- If you feel that you have somehow side-stepped your life's calling, that something profound is missing, that your life or your job is like a pair of gloves that have never felt as though they fit you quite right, just know it doesn't have to be that way.

- If you feel that you have not fully developed your natural talents and abilities, have no opportunity to use them, or believe you have no natural talents or abilities whatsoever, just know it doesn't have to be that way.

My primary focus right now is to help you identify and erase the causes and effects of professional burnout and assist in transforming your life by helping to:

- Restore the joy and happiness you once felt in the everyday practice of medicine.
- Identify and develop your true inner passions.
- Identify, develop and employ your natural talents and abilities for purposeful work.
- Positively remodel your mind-set and fine tune it for success.
- Unleash your creative potential.
- Assess the health and needs of all four of your personal realms — the mental, emotional, physical, and spiritual realms.

Have these goals in mind as you proceed through this workbook.

What are your specific goals? What do you wish to accomplish? Make a list of them here.

_____
_____
_____
_____
_____
_____
_____
_____

The REIGNITE Workbook

Setting the Stage: A Bit of the History of Medicine

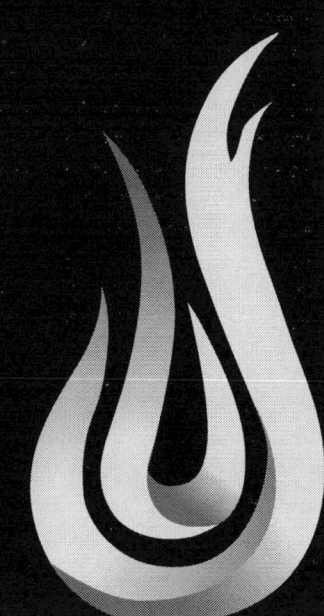

Do you know who this might be?

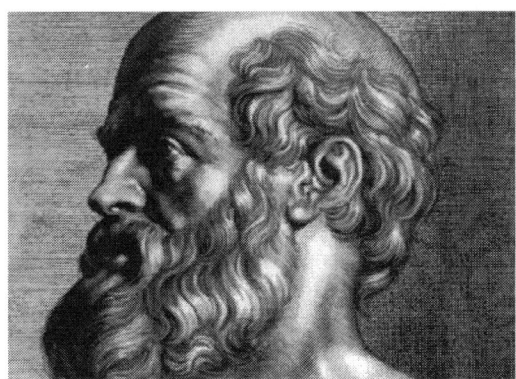

This engraving is by Peter Paul Rubens, 1638. The answer is on the next page.

This is Hippocrates, our Greek father of Western medicine, circa 460 – circa 370 BC. He began the Hippocratic School of Medicine which revolutionized the practice of medicine in ancient Greece. It was his discipline that established medicine as a distinct profession. It is in his name that we swear our oath to, among other things, first do no harm.

Does this person look familiar to you?

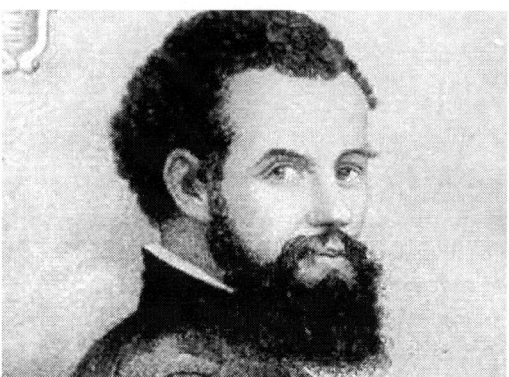

This notable gave us our first glimpse into what makes us tick. Again, the answer is on the following page.

He is Andreas Vesalius, 1514 – 1564, the father of human anatomy. He was the first to systematically dissect the human body and record what he saw. The result was the book On the Fabric of the Human Body, one of the most influential texts in medicine ever written.

How about this woman? Does she ring any bells?

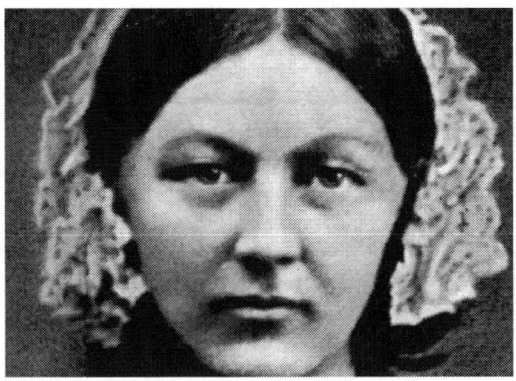

She lived from 1820 to 1910 and taught all of us in medicine some very important lessons.

Right you are! It's Florence Nightingale, the mother of the modern nursing profession. She began a school of nursing which established nursing as a profession. She was also a social reformer and her healthcare reforms touched nearly every aspect of British Society. International Nurses Day is celebrated annually around the world on her birthday.

Would you know the name of this rather stern looking woman?

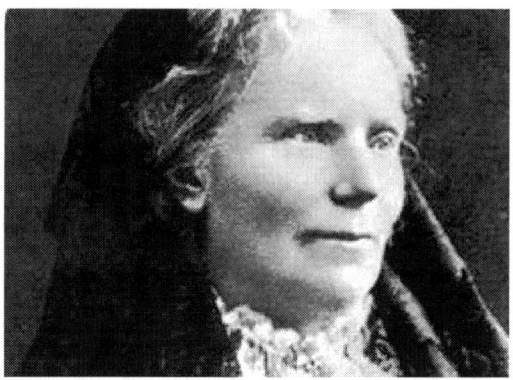

She broke glass ceilings before they called them glass ceilings.

This is Elizabeth Blackwell, 1821 – 1910. She was the first woman to receive a medical degree in the United States and a pioneer for promoting the education of women in medicine. She was also a social and moral reformer. Her sister, Emily, was the third woman in the United States to earn a medical degree.

Care to hazard a guess as to the identity of this Union Army solider?

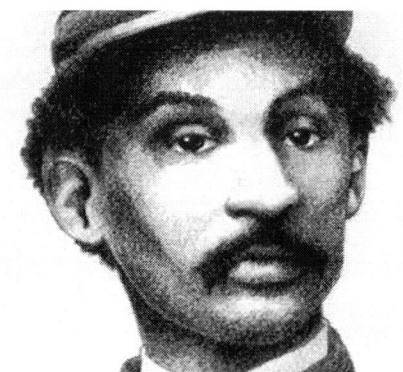

He served with distinction in the Union Army and at the bedside of a dying man who's name you will know. Although few people know the name of this man. If you do, you are quite the historian!

This is Dr. Anderson Ruffin Abbott, 1837 – 1913. He was the first black Canadian to become a licensed physician. He petitioned Abraham Lincoln to join the Union Army and he rose through the ranks with distinguished service, one of only thirteen black surgeons to serve in the Civil War. After Lincoln was shot, Dr. Abbott attended Lincoln's deathbed. Mary Todd Lincoln was so moved by his devotion that she gave him the plaid shawl that Lincoln wore to his 1861 inaugural. Dr. Abbott wore it to Lincoln's funeral.

Surely, you know the name of this man.

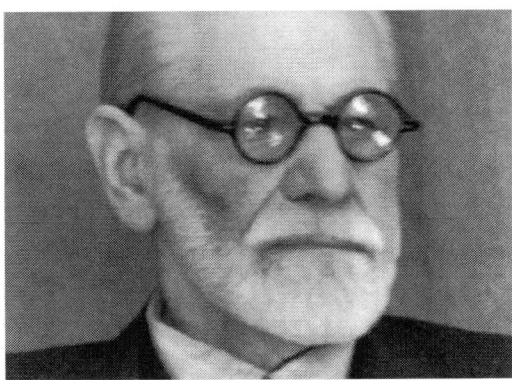

Hint: He was able to describe how screwed up we all are and why.

Correct! It's Sigmund Freud, 1856 – 1939, the Father of Psychoanalysis. Free association, transference, the Oedipus Complex, libido, the theory of the unconscious, and the death drive — all theories that we owe to the good Dr. Freud.

Do you know the men in this painting entitled The Four Doctors?

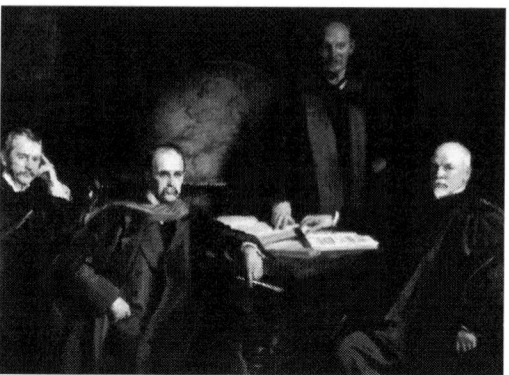

It was painted by John Singer Sargent and completed in 1906. From the left are William Welch, William Halsted, Sir William Osler and Howard Kelly. All are famous but especially Sir William Osler, who is the acknowledged father of modern medicine. These four doctors started Johns Hopkins Hospital.

There is a point to all of this, I promise. Last but not least, who might this be?

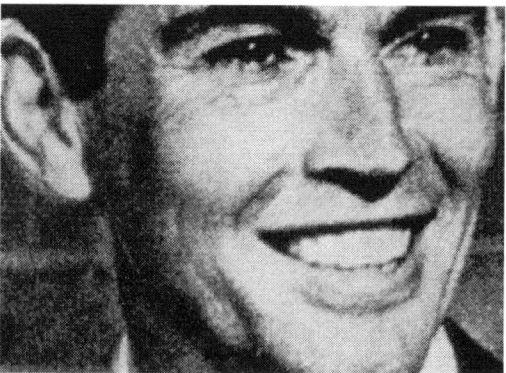

He had a thing for kidneys and hearts.

This man is Christian Barnard, 1922 – 2001. Dr. Barnard performed the second ever kidney transplant in South Africa in 1967.

He, of course, went on to perform the first human-to-human heart transplant on December 3, 1967. Assisted by his brother, Dr. Marius Barnard, the operation lasted nine hours and required a team of thirty people. He studied medicine up until the day he died.

All of these great men and women in medicine have one thing in common and one thing only. Care to guess what that might be?

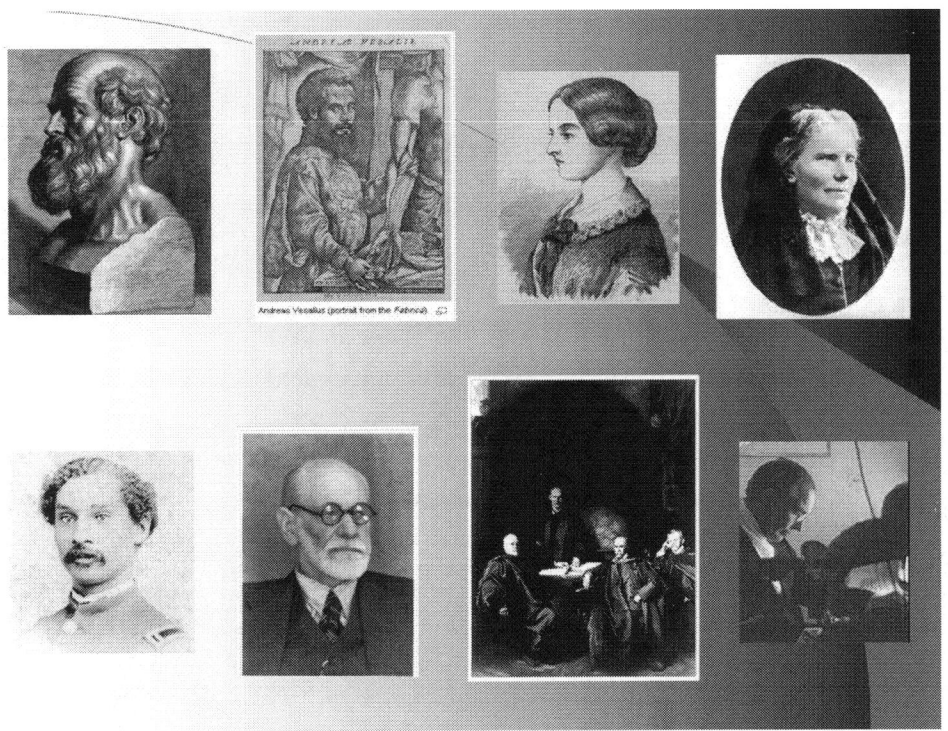

The answer may surprise you. But, all of these great women and men in medicine are…

dead. Dead, dead, dead, dead, DEAD! Not only are they dead, all of their patients are dead.

I don't know about you, but I got into medicine to save lives. Many of you reading this material probably did as well. Well, one night while working the ICU during residency training and about two weeks into my Internal Medicine rotation, I had what amounts to a life enlightening epiphany. You can not save the same life over and over and over again.

No one lives forever. No one will make it out of this life alive. We all eventually lose that battle with our patients and ultimately ourselves. So, what is it that we do in medicine? What can we offer our patients? What hope can we give them? What hope can we retain for ourselves?

Of course, for our patients, our first charge is do no harm. Beyond that, we strive to eliminate pain and suffering, help our patients to extend their lives, and make it a better quality of life if we can. If we can help our patients extend that which is most precious, life, by giving them more time in this world to do what they wish to do, then we have done our job well for them and the house of medicine. This should be your source for a great deal of satisfaction in the practice of medicine.

I can think of no more noble a gift than to give our patients more time on this Earth, especially if it is years they can enjoy. It is an extremely sad occurrence when physicians burn out and come to feel they do not make this difference in their patients' lives anymore.

Do you feel that you still make a difference in the lives of your patients?

Moreover, our own life is short, fleeting. Too precious to waste feeling miserable. Like those great men and women in medicine, you want to make a contribution. You want to make a difference in the lives of your patients. At the same time, you want to enjoy the full richness of what life has to offer. Am I right about this?

Has this become a task too difficult or a seemingly impossible balance to strike for you?   YES   or   NO

It is a national shame that so many of our experienced physicians are facing the professional malady known as burnout. Physicians spend so much time, energy and resource educating themselves and training that it is a personal tragedy when one leaves the workforce due to something completely preventable and treatable such as job-related burnout.

The nation, states and local communities also invest a tremendous amount of resources to attract and retain good doctors. The costs associated with becoming a physician are fast becoming prohibitively expensive. It does the public a great disservice to lose such vital expertise.

Actual direct costs to replace a physician can cost practices and organizations between $150,000.00 and $1,000,000.00+ due to expenses related to recruiting, contracting, start-up, lost revenue generation, advertising, etc. Indirect costs can be just as high.

It is incumbent on individual physicians, or the practices and groups that hire them, to do whatever they can to prevent burnout, alleviate the symptoms of burnout or treat burnout by taking appropriate actions as soon as possible.

There are plans, strategies and programs that can easily be put into place, which will lessen or eliminate the impact of healthcare provider burnout.

In the next section, we will begin to talk about happiness in the everyday practice of medicine.

Defining Happiness in the Practice of Medicine

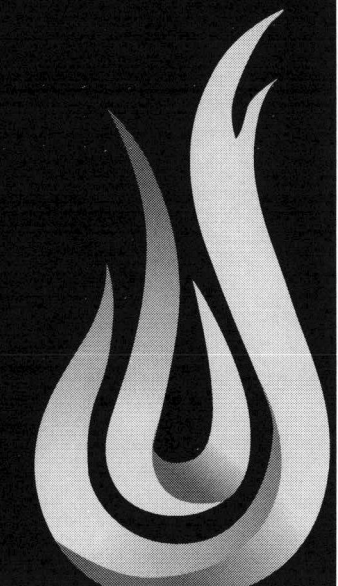

What is your happiness quotient, Doctor? Are you serenely happy? Or, perfectly broken? Are you living an engaged life or merely existing and feeling detached? What is the overall, big-picture state of your being?

Happiness, like beauty, is in the eye of the beholder. The definition of happiness in the everyday practice of medicine will be different for different providers.

For instance, for one physician happiness may mean less pressure to crank through large numbers of patients in a single day. To another physician happiness might mean getting to work more with a particular patient type and less with another patient type.

Happiness may not be the absence of problems. We deal with patient problems all day. What would we do were it not for problems to solve? How you handle everyday problems and difficulties may be more of a determinant of how happy or unhappy you are.

Still, for most physicians, I believe happiness in the everyday practice of medicine would likely be associated with a longer list of positives rather than an absence of negatives. Today, I believe most of the unhappiness in the practice of medicine to be more closely associated with a paucity of positives and an ever-expanding list of negatives.

Choosing to accentuate the positives or amplify the negatives of one's work in the practice of medicine has everything to do with one's mindset. The burned out mindset is a reflection of severe job dissatisfaction, plain and simple. How do physicians end up this way?

Just as in any relationship or marriage, there is the ideal mate and then there is the one you end with or marry. If you laughed at the truth in this statement, just remember that your partner would probably do the same thing. (:-D)

In the practice of medicine, there is the ideal practice and then there is your current practice reality. Are the two images in your head right now radically different? If so, what changed? If they are radically different, it can't all just be on-the-job stress. The ideal stress-free practice is a myth — an illusion.

Remember when you were in medical school, how hard it was, how stressful it was but also how exciting at the same time? Then, there was the expectancy of entering the clinical rotations. I remember how I was both scared and thrilled to finally be working with patients.

Remember how proud and happy you were to begin your residency training? Perhaps then, in your last year of training, there was the planning and search for the kind of practice you envisioned for yourself and the dreams of the life you would provide for your family.

I can still remember my first day in private practice on Monday August 3rd, 1992. I was so excited! All those years of hard work and sacrifice would culminate on that day at 8:30 a.m. Do you remember your first day in practice? What that felt like?

If you are reading this now, over the ensuing years, that feeling of exhilaration has probably been replaced by a sense of dread. You may be experiencing some of the symptoms of burnout, well on your way to burnout, or already in full-blown burnout. How did this happen?

There is a culture of medicine that has been idealized and personified from many different directions, entities and personalities. There was little regard for doctors at the turn of the twentieth century. It wasn't until medical education was formalized and the medical licensing boards came into existence that doctors of medicine gained credibility and respectability. Medicine became a science.

Over many years, the field of medicine became the epitome of professional careers. The doctor became a symbol for many superlatives including healing, comfort, empathy, success, long suffering, self-sacrifice, intelligence, humanitarianism, virtue, and perfection. Not all of that was deserved. Somewhere in the mix, the word human got lost.

Nowhere were these notions of what a doctor was, or should be, portrayed more idealistically and romantically than in TV and film.

The Public's Perception of the Good Doctor

If you have some age on you, you may well remember Dr. Ben Casey (Vince Edwards).

The REIGNITE Workbook

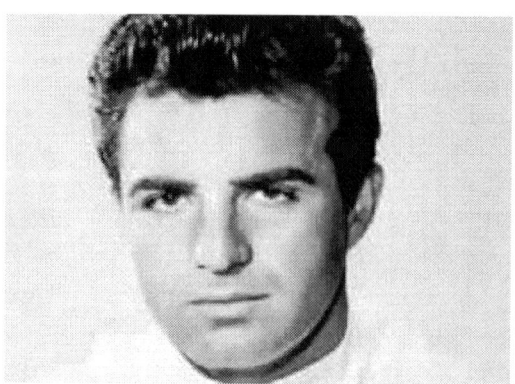

This was a television medical drama series that ran on ABC from 1961 – 1966. The show became know for its opening titles, which consisted of a hand drawing out the symbols ♂ ♀ * † ∞ on a chalk board as cast member Dr. David Zorba (Sam Jaffe) in a low voice intoned, "man, woman, birth, death, infinity." It was all very dramatically done.

Dr. David Zorba.

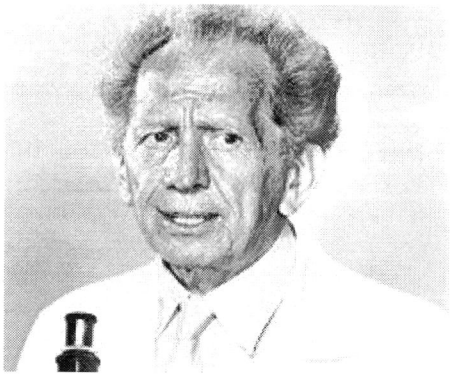

A neurosurgeon, Dr. Joseph Ransohoff, was a medical consultant for the show and may have influenced the personality of Dr. Ben Casey, the title character.

Then, there was every young woman's heart throb, Dr. Kildare, played by Richard Chamberlain. This was another very popular medical drama TV series from 1961 – 1966.

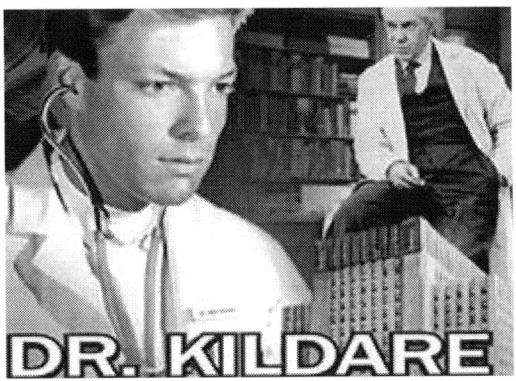

Almost everyone with ten years of practice or more under their belt can recall the medical TV drama Marcus Welby, MD. It aired from September 1961 to July 1976. Robert Young played Marcus Welby. Everybody wanted a doctor like Dr. Marcus Welby. Every would-be doctor wanted to be like Dr. Marcus Welby. As you can see below, this show is still popular as the series is now offered in DVD format.

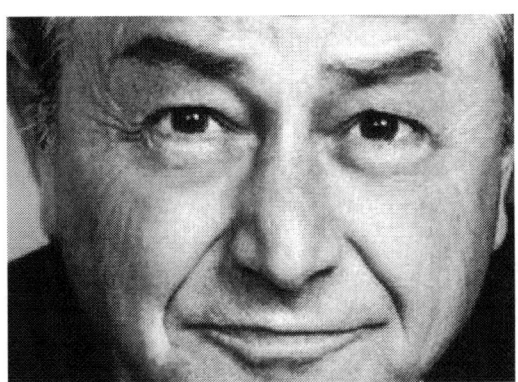

It is both interesting and tragic to note, Robert Young's life was anything but the happy and well-adjusted persona portrayed in his television series. He suffered from depression and alcoholism, which led to a suicide attempt seven years before his death from respiratory failure at the age of ninety-one. How many physicians out there, who appear to be leading happy and well-adjusted, lives are in turmoil and suffering on the inside? No one knows for sure.

You may be too young to remember these romanticized television portrayals of what a physician's life and practice were like. If so, that's okay. Just know that these early television shows, and the ones that followed them, helped to shape the country's perception of what medical practices were like and what the doctors who worked in them were like.

Guess what? If you are old enough to remember these shows, then they shaped your perceptions, the perceptions of those of us who ended up in medicine, no less. Along with these perceptions came a whole boatload of expectations! Some were based in reality. A fair amount were not.

Medical training fostered and perpetuated the notion of the lone eagle, long-suffering, non-complaining, perfectionist physician who sees to everyone's needs with little regard for his own. Physicians were taught to suck it up, even when sick. In fact, illness came to be regarded as weakness.

Where are you on the Happiness Continuum

What is your happiness quotient, Doctor? Are you serenely happy? Or, perfectly broken? Are you living and engaged or merely existing and feeling detached? What is the overall, big-picture state of your being?

_____
_____
_____
_____
_____

The Ideal Versus the Reality

In the practice of medicine, there is the ideal practice and then there is your current practice reality. Are the two images in your head right now radically different? If so, what changed? Describe the difference.

_____
_____
_____
_____

Growing up, was there someone you wanted to emulate by becoming a physician? Was there a mentor you looked up to while in training? Do you think your career in medicine unfolded differently from theirs? How so?

_____
_____
_____
_____

What would make you happy right now?

If you are reading this material, it is probably safe to say that you are currently unhappy with the practice of medicine, your life overall, or both. Most likely you are burning out or close to being burned out. There are always contributing factors.

It will be quite instructional for you to compile a list of items that you feel are contributing to your feelings of burnout. It could be one item or many.

Take a moment and list those items. List anything and everything you would change or feel is missing from your life, which if changed, eliminated or acquired would make you happy or happier right now. This can be within the practice of medicine or outside of it.

Defining Burnout

How does one define physician burnout? There are many different ways but only one best way to define burnout. Here are some currently accepted definitions.

Mosby's Medical Dictionary 2009 defines burnout thus:
A popular term for a mental or physical energy depletion after a period of chronic, unrelieved job stress characterized sometimes by physical illness. The person suffering from burnout may lose concern or respect for other people and often has cynical, dehumanized perceptions of people, labeling them in a derogatory manner.

An emotional condition marked by tiredness, loss of interest, or frustration that interferes with job performance. Burnout is usually regarded as the result of prolonged stress.

Mosby's Dictionary of Complementary and Alternative Medicine 2005 defines burnout as:
1. a state that occurs when energy is used up faster than it is restored.
2. psychological and physical fatigue of a caregiver resulting in apathy and depression.

The Miller-Keane Encyclopedia and Dictionary of Medicine, Nursing and Allied Health, Seventh Edition 2003 gives the definition of burnout as:

Emotional and physical exhaustion resulting from a combination of exposure to environmental and internal stressors and inadequate coping and adaptive skills. In addition to signs of exhaustion, the person with burnout exhibits an increasingly negative attitude toward his or her job, low self-esteem, and personal devaluation.

Notice all of the characteristics each of these definitions have in common.

The Industry Standard Definition – The MBI

The best and most accurate definition of burnout would enable one to quantify it in a way that is both sensitive and specific. This brings us to the seminal work published in 1981 by Christina Maslach and Susan E. Jackson entitled **The measurement of experienced burnout.**

This was the work that defined burnout with the creation of an instrument for measuring the various aspects of the burnout syndrome. This led to the development of the Maslach Burnout Inventory (MBI), an assessment tool that is still valid and in widely accepted use today.

The authors discovered three defining hallmarks of physician (or professional) burnout. The three hallmarks of burnout are:

- **Emotional Exhaustion** – Measures feelings of being emotionally overextended and exhausted by one's work. This is a feeling of being so emotionally depleted you're at a point where you feel you can no longer give of yourself at an emotional or psychological level. You feel you just have nothing more to give. **Keyword: EXHAUSTION**
- **Depersonalization** – Measures an unfeeling and impersonal response toward recipients of one's service, care/treatment or instruction. Negative and cynical feelings are developed leading to a callous and dehumanized perception of patients, clients or customers, which further leads to the view that they are somehow deserving of their problems and troubles. **Keyword: CYNICISM**
- **Lack of a Sense of Personal Accomplishment** – Measures feelings of competence and successful achievement in one's work. The physician feels so little reward there is a tendency to evaluate oneself in negative terms, which leads to dissatisfaction and unhappiness in one's work. This creates a lack of a sense of personal accomplishment. **Keyword: INEFFICACY**

The reasons job-related burnout (JRB) develops is multifactorial and the order in which the hallmarks appear are different for men and women.

Burnout in Women

Women tend to hit each of the hallmarks of burnout as they are presented above — **Emotional Exhaustion** followed by **Depersonalization** followed by a **Lack of a Sense of Personal Accomplishment.**

The emergence of emotional exhaustion should serve as an early warning sign that burnout has begun. As with most things, the symptoms of burnout are most easily alleviated early once the underlying causes are properly identified and addressed.

Women may become depressed or act out in maladaptive and self-destructive ways once they have progressed through all three stages of burnout.

Women who progress through all three stages will leave medicine altogether if no action is taken to address the underlying causes of their burnout.

Burnout in Men

Men typically develop **Depersonalization** first with the emergence of cynicism. This is usually employed as a coping mechanism for overwhelming stress and signals the early development of burnout.

Emotional Exhaustion comes next and this is when many male healthcare providers can begin to act out in various maladaptive and self-destructive ways. Excessive alcohol intake; self-medication with narcotics, benzodiazepines and/or illicit drugs; aberrant behavioral diversions such as gambling addiction, sex addiction, extramarital affairs, and patient boundary violations are all common attempts to alter the mood and reduce stress.

Unlike women, men almost never reach a complete **Lack of a Sense of Personal Accomplishment**. Men will not often see or admit emotional exhaustion and depersonalization as something affecting their work. They will continue to view themselves as a good doctor despite their cynicism and emotional exhaustion, which is usually readily apparent to everyone around them. For this reason, they will continue to practice in a perpetual state of burnout, which causes perpetual unhappiness.

Stress Versus Burnout

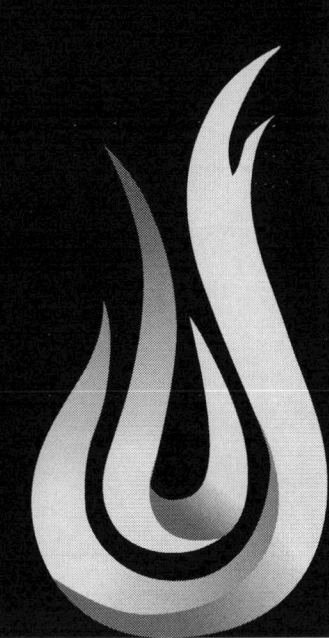

Everyone feels stressed at times. Stress, when not excessive, can be healthy. It can keep us on our toes, conscientious, sharp, alert, on time, motivated and moving forward. It is when stress becomes excessive and transitions to distress that it becomes toxic.

Physicians are people too, just like everyone else. Just like everyone else, physicians face a lot of stressors and dis-stressors such as uncertainty in the workplace, overextension (time commitments, debt, work, etc.), feeling a loss of control, personal health issues, relationship issues, a seminal event that is out of proportion to everyday experience (tragedy), a preponderance of small stressors, perfect storm scenarios…the list goes ever on. You, of course, know best of all what stresses you out.

Oh yes, I forgot to mention the biggest stressor of all — FEAR. An endless parade of fears, like the fear of making a mistake, losing patients, being sued, missing something, killing someone, not being liked, failing in the business aspect of medicine, flagging income, increased scrutiny and on and on.

Dr. Hans Selye, an endocrinologist, did extensive research on physiologic stress back in the 1940s and 50s. He posited that overt stress had two components, a set of normal responses he called the general adaptation syndrome and the development of a pathologic state from persistent, unremitting stress.

This pathologic state encompasses the toxic nature of burnout. He classified three stages in the development of maladaptive stress.

- **Alarm is the first stage.** When the threat or stressor is identified or realized, the body's stress response is in a state of alarm. During this stage, adrenaline is produced in order to invoke the fight or flight response. Except now days, you can't fight and you can't flee from what transpires on the job, no matter how bad your day becomes. Although, some days you probably wish you could do precisely that.
- **Resistance is the second stage.** If the stressor(s) persist, some means becomes necessary to cope with the stress. The mind and body will try to compensate and adapt to the strains and demands of the work environment but are unable to keep this up indefinitely. So, the body's compensatory mechanisms and resources gradually deplete.
- **Exhaustion is the third and final stage.** At this point, all of the body's coping resources are depleted and unable to maintain normal function. If stage three is extended over a long period of time, damage may result as the mind and body become exhausted. Normal function becomes impaired resulting in decompensation.

Although stress is a contributor to burnout, it is just one of many causes and factors associated with burnout. They are not one and the same. You can be stressed out but not burned out. But, if you are burned out I can say with 100% assurance that you are stressed or distressing.

Therefore, it is important to note that although stress reduction strategies may offer some real benefit, they will not alleviate all of the symptoms of burnout because stress is not the only cause.

There are many differences between stress and burnout. Here are some of those differences:

- Stress is characterized by over-engagement. Burnout is characterized by disengagement.
- In stress emotions are overactive. In burnout emotions are blunted.
- Stress produces urgency and hyperactivity. Burnout produces helplessness and hopelessness.
- Stress leads to loss of energy. Burnout leads to loss of motivation, ideals and hope.
- Stress leads to anxiety disorders. Burnout leads to detachment and depression.
- With stress the damage is primarily physical. With burnout the damage is primarily emotional.
- Stress may kill you prematurely. Burnout will make life seem not worth living and increases your risk of suicide. Burnout makes you feel like you are dead already.
- Stress is more easily identified and treated. Full-blown burnout can be much more difficult to manage as it includes stress and many other factors.
- Stress is almost always recognized by the individual. Burnout may not be recognized as such by the individual. Symptoms may be incorrectly attributed to some other cause, such as stress.

What are some of the **stressors** you feel may be contributing to your symptoms of burnout? These can be on-the-job stressors or come from outside of work. List them here:

_____   _____
_____   _____
_____   _____
_____   _____
_____   _____
_____   _____
_____   _____
_____   _____
_____   _____
_____   _____
_____   _____
_____   _____
_____   _____

The Causes of Job-Related Burnout

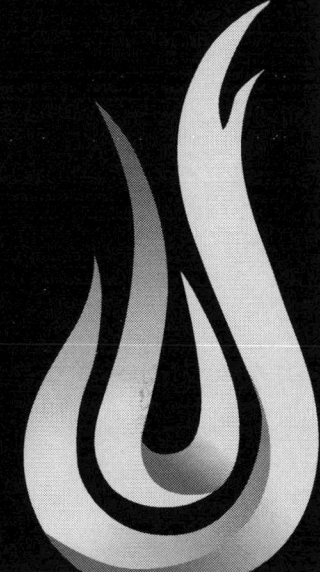

Physicians must work in highly emotionally active and reactive situations often associated with suffering, fear, trepidation, failures, disease and death. These situations often culminate in difficult interactions with patients, families and other medical personnel. At the same time, we wish to be trusted and viewed favorably by our patients, peers and community.

Additionally, rapid changes to the practice of medicine — such as increased patient care demands, reimbursement issues, expanding healthcare bureaucracy, increased accountability measures, and conflict between the needs of healthcare systems and those of patients — are all threats to physician health and wellness.

You can not, **CAN NOT**, be a healthcare provider and be unaffected by all of this. As stressors mount, physicians may find themselves ill equipped to adjust professionally and personally.

Unaddressed or unresolved stress can lead to unresolved anger. Unresolved anger leads to increasing resentments. Unresolved resentments lead inexorably to fractured relationships at work, at home or both, which just makes matters worse.

Burnout can develop insidiously over many years. It can be the slow drip of a preponderance of little frustrations that sum up over time — frustrations shoved into the background because they seem small or insignificant at the time, something better to be dealt with "later."

All of this frustration and emotional pain is kept inside until at some point, a seemingly innocuous trigger can cause it to all come flooding out. To those looking on, it seems as though there was some kind of acute break. The truth is, **burnout is the end of a process, not the beginning of one.**

Individuals who burn out the **fastest** have at least one or all of the following — onerous or adversarial work environments, lives that are out of balance, poor coping skills, lack of resilience, inability to voice their feelings, no clear sense of who they are or what they want, an addiction, undiagnosed or untreated depression, or are facing multiple tragic circumstances over which they feel they have no control.

Sounds harsh, I know. But none of these issues are insurmountable. They can all be addressed and overcome with intentional effort.

If you were to list items you feel are causing symptoms of burnout, what would they be? They may be the same, similar or different to other items you have previously listed in this workbook. But try not to think about those right now.

Common Causes of Provider Burnout

Here is a partial list of some of the most common causes of healthcare provider burnout. If any of these feel familiar or directly apply to you, circle them or add them to your written list.

Lack of peer support
Perfectionism
The compulsion to prove oneself
Inadequate pay/reimbursement
Neglecting own needs
Compromise of core values/value conflicts
Working harder to compensate for failures or inadequacies
Ever increasing bureaucratic demands
Hypercritical administrators
Lack of recognition
Tasks with no apparent end
Lack of autonomy
Conflicting roles at work and at home
Meaninglessness of achieved goals (success burnout)
Nearly impossible tasks requiring solutions/overwhelmed
Difficult or unappreciative clients or patients
Inner emptiness
Poor health
Overextended with time commitments
Overburdened with debt requiring more hours of work
No interest outside of medicine/work
Healthcare/Medicine not a good career fit for personality
Social and emotional skills deficits
Sense of an utter lack of control
Little time off
Inadequate rest
Too little time with patients

I want you to list here anything and everything else you feel might be contributing to your symptoms of **burnout**, even items not related to work

_____   _____
_____   _____
_____   _____
_____   _____
_____   _____
_____   _____
_____   _____
_____   _____
_____   _____
_____   _____
_____   _____
_____   _____
_____   _____
_____   _____

The Signs and Symptoms of Burnout

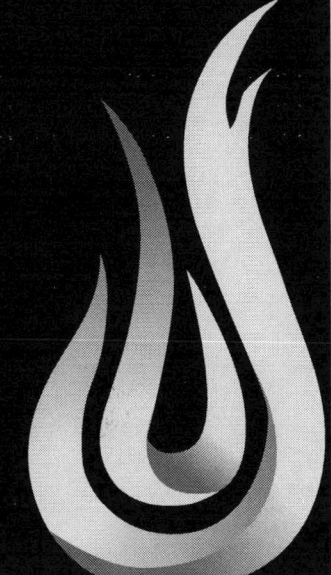

First and foremost, the signs and symptoms of physician burnout are eminently identified, amenable to treatment, and wholly preventable. For physicians already suffering from the effects of JRB, just know that it doesn't have to be that way.

The signs and symptoms of burnout can be subtle to overt. Its development is a gradual process, usually over an extended period of time. Unless the underlying causes are identified, addressed and corrected, burnout tends to get progressively worse over time for most people. If full-blown burnout occurs, the consequences can be severe and very difficult to reverse.

The following realms are affected by burnout, and some of the salient signs and symptoms of each are listed.

- **Mental Signs** – Inability to concentrate, short-term memory impairment, cognitive impairment, easily distracted, difficulty making simple decisions.

- **Physical Signs** – Feeling tired, lethargic, or sick quite often. Decreased appetite and/or sleep disturbance. Frequent headaches, dizziness, back pain, muscle aches.
- **Emotional Signs** – Feeling detached and lonely. An overwhelming sense of failure or self-doubt. Feeling helpless, trapped, or defeated. Loss of motivation. An increasingly cynical and pessimistic outlook. A lack of a sense of accomplishment in life. Lack of empathy. Anger, impatience, irritability.
- **Spiritual Signs** – A profound dissatisfaction with oneself, others, the world and of living. Unsourced and unnamed fears and anxieties. Unreal feelings that can not be described. Feeling as though you are living outside of your true self. An unrest or unease deep inside that can not be adequately described. Feeling empty.
- **Behavioral Signs** – Withdrawing from people and responsibilities. Isolating, procrastinating and avoidance behaviors. Unprofessional behavior. Use of food, drugs, alcohol or addictive behaviors as a coping mechanism. Increased irritability and lashing out at others. Skipping out on work or working at odd hours.

What seems to be the matter, Doctor?

Ask yourself the following questions. Please, circle all which apply to you.

Do you find you are:

More time pressured?	YES	NO
Less patient?	YES	NO
More irritable/angry?	YES	NO
Less empathetic?	YES	NO
More intolerant?	YES	NO
Less enthusiastic?	YES	NO
More exhausted?	YES	NO
More cynical?	YES	NO
Less and less in control?	YES	NO
Doubtful of your abilities?	YES	NO
Doubtful of your career choice?	YES	NO
Considering an early retirement?	YES	NO
No longer recommending medicine as a profession?	YES	NO

Are there others you could add to this list?

_____
_____
_____
_____
_____
_____
_____

If you get the sense that you are developing the symptoms of burnout, or if you feel that you are burned out, I would suggest you proceed with taking the Maslach Burnout Inventory (MBI) questionnaire and continue working through the material in this workbook.

The Scope of Physician Burnout

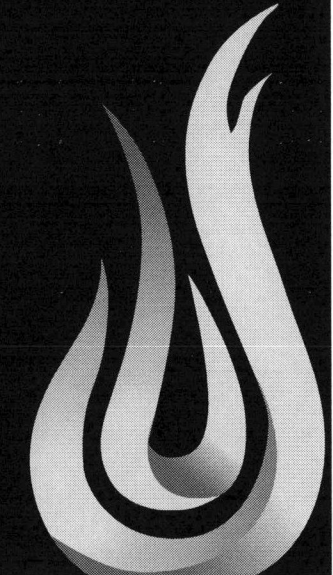

I f you are feeling burned out, you are not alone!

Physician burnout is more than a growing concern in the United States, it is an epidemic. While burnout rates may vary among the myriad medical specialties, that in no way reduces the impact associated with each of them, nor does it lessen the risks involved. All demographic groups are affected.

Among the nation's healthcare providers, burnout rates can approach 70% in some specialties. If not properly addressed, this can lead to immense dissatisfaction within the practice of medicine or a loss of expertise through early retirement, an alternate career choice, or acting out through addiction to alcohol, drugs or other addictive behaviors.

The house of medicine is literally on fire and the physicians are the ones burning. In my opinion, physician burnout is a NATIONAL EMERGENCY.

The Statistics:

The facts are in, and it is very clear that we have a big problem when it comes to physicians experiencing burnout in this country. Burnout among physicians is worse than among other professional workers, and it has been a catastrophe in the making for some time now. Here are some of the numbers:

- In 1987, an AMA survey showed that 44% of physician respondents over the age of forty would not choose medicine as a career if they had it to do all over again.
- A 2001 survey of physicians in Massachusetts found 62.3% dissatisfied with their practice environment.
- A survey by the Kaiser Family Foundation in 2002 revealed that 45% of physicians would not recommend that a young person choose medicine as a career choice.
- A 2007 survey of primary care physicians found 38.7% were somewhat or very dissatisfied with the practice of medicine.
- A 2011 survey of 2,069 physicians by Physician Wellness Services, a Minneapolis based company, found 87% of respondents felt moderately or severely stressed or burned out daily. The median age was forty-five with an average of thirteen years in practice.
- In a survey that was presented to 13,000 physicians in 2012, six out of ten physicians would quit today if financially able to do so. That's 60%!
- A 2012 study of 7,288 physicians published in the Archives of Internal Medicine revealed that 46% reported at least one symptom of burnout.
- From an Academic Medicine paper dated July 2012, 14%

of respondents had seriously considered leaving their own institution during the prior year and 21% had seriously considered leaving academic medicine altogether due to dissatisfaction.
- Burnout rates approach 70% in some specialties. Specialties with higher than average rates of burnout were Emergency Medicine, Family Medicine, General Internal Medicine, and Neurology.
- The highest burnout rates for physicians are in the specialties of Emergency Medicine and Critical Care.
- One report shows that nearly 50% of practicing radiologists surveyed had at least one symptom of burnout.
- The burnout rate among female physicians at 60% is higher than the male physician burnout rate of 52%.
- Burnout rates are highest in the forty-six to fifty-five age bracket.
- Using the Primary Care Evaluation of Mental Disorders screening instrument, the percentage of depressed physicians who may have been depressed was 37.8%, much higher than the national average across the general population.
- Suicide rates among physicians are significantly higher, six times higher, than the rate in the general population. Having a job problem that contributed to suicide significantly predicted the likelihood of being a physician.
- A Medscape survey found that although physicians in the specialty of OB/GYN and Women's Health did not rank themselves highest in terms of percentage of physicians burned out, they did rank their burnout as the most severe compared to other specialties.
- Cardiovascular mortality is higher among physicians.
- Up to 14% of practicing physicians have or will develop a substance abuse problem, higher than the national average.
- Burnout doesn't just affect US physicians. In a 2013 study, 82% of Chinese physicians said that they were burned out compared to 42% of US physicians.
- In the December 2015 issue of Mayo Clinic Proceedings, a

study by Shanafelt, et. al. documented a rapid rise in burnout rates experienced by US physicians. Using the Maslach Burnout Inventory assessment tool, burnout rates rose from 45.5% in 2011 to 54.4% in 2014, a rise of 8.9% in just three years. The study's conclusion — More than half of all US physicians are now experiencing professional burnout!

So it goes, on and on and on. This is a problem that is getting relatively little attention and it's getting much worse!

At the Global Forum of Health Leaders in Taipei, Taiwan, Dana Hanson, President of the World Medical Association spoke about "silent desperation" among some doctors adding, "many were inwardly burning."

Dr. Hanson and others have concluded that healthy doctors meant healthier patients, safer care and a more sustainable workforce. Dr. Hanson went further stating, "Physicians should not have to choose between saving themselves and serving their patients."

"Six out of ten physicians would quit today if financially able to do so."

This is an astounding, no, a shocking statistic!

Here is a worse one.

In one study, 90% of practicing physicians surveyed said they would not recommend medicine as a career path to a familymember.

The way you feel right now, would you recommend medicine as a career path to a friend or family member?   YES   or   NO

Is It Our Profession's Fault?

From the Accreditation Council for Graduate Medical Education (ACGME) comes this statement — Residents must demonstrate *"a responsiveness to patient needs that supersedes self-interest."* This statement is profound in that it requires physicians in training to learn self-sacrifice as part of professional identity.

Inculcating physicians with the notion that self-care is secondary to all else is pervasive within the house of medicine. Physicians who are struggling, addicted or sick are loath to reach out to colleagues for help for fear of being viewed as weak somehow.

In residency training we were expected to function normally after working long and exhausting hours. Any complaint was likely to be met with something from the attending or chief resident like "suck it up," "you don't have it half as bad as I did when I was a resident," or "asking for help is a sign of weakness."

Attitudes in some training programs are beginning to change but not fast enough. A specific course on stress management, burnout, wellness and life balance needs to be offered or, better yet, required in residency training.

Try to be completely honest as you answer the following questions.

Have you ever worked while sick? Circle one: YES   or   NO

Have you ever viewed a sick colleague as being weak somehow?
Circle one: YES   or   NO

After hearing of a colleague who has taken time off from work for an acute illness, have you ever thought, "I've been sicker than that before and I came on in and worked anyway"?

Circle one: YES   or   NO

Have you ever felt guilty for taking needed time away or off from work?

Circle one: YES   or   NO

Assessing Burnout: The Maslach Burnout Inventory (MBI)

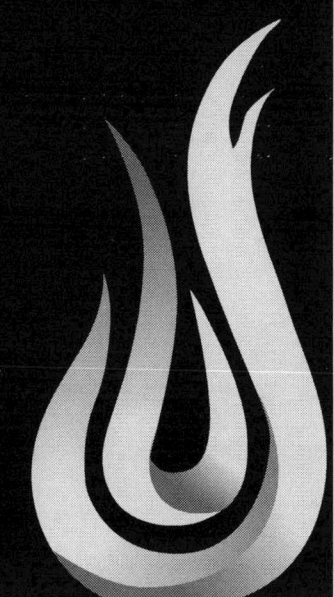

The Maslach Burnout Inventory developed by Christina Maslach, et. al., is an industry standard measurement tool for assessing burnout in the human services arena. As such, it lends itself very well to assessing burnout amongst physicians and other healthcare providers where the results have meaningful application.

The MBI is considered the gold standard in measuring physician burnout.

The MBI consists of a twenty-two-item questionnaire that measures burnout with sensitivity, specificity and reproducibility. Questions in the MBI measure both the frequency and intensity of feelings.

Here is a sample MBI question and accompanying response list:

I feel used up at the end of the workday.

    0 - Never
    1 - A few times a year or less
    2 - Once a month or less
    3 - A few times a month
    4 - Once a week
    5 - A few times a week
    6 - Every day

There are nine items in the **Emotional Exhaustion** subscale, five items in the **Depersonalization** subscale and eight items in the **Personal Accomplishment** subscale.

Scores for each physician or healthcare provider can be coded as low, average or high for each subscale. This enables every respondent to compare themselves to the overall prevailing norms. Each individual can gauge their own experience with the hallmarks of burnout.

Original numeric scores can be used in aggregate for statistical analysis. This is a powerful tool for large groups or organizations. Comparing MBI scores before intervention with scores after intervention programs have been implemented can provide accurate measures of efficacy.

If you feel you may be experiencing the signs and symptoms of burnout, you should definitely self-assess by taking the MBI. The MBI is offered once as part of this instructional course on physician burnout.

If at any point you wish to reassess, an additional MBI can be purchased separately here for comparison scoring.

What Is the State Opposite of Burnout?

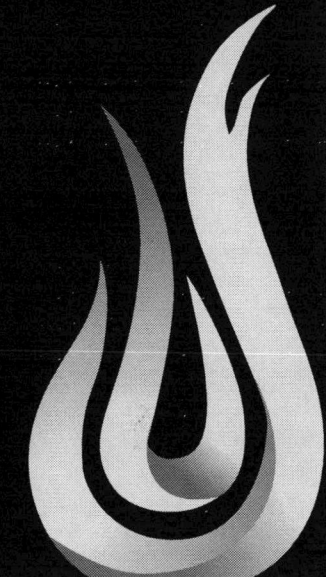

I have described in a great deal of detail the nature of job-related burnout, its causes, the scope of burnout and how it is assessed.

If you will recall, the burnout syndrome is three dimensional with the salient features of exhaustion, cynicism and inefficacy. If burnout represents all that is undesirable about the practice of one's profession (medicine), what is its antithesis? In short, what is the human state opposite of burnout?

In a word, it's **ENGAGEMENT**.

Engagement is an energetic state in which an individual is dedicated to excellent performance at work with confidence in their effectiveness. To be engaged is to be completely present in your work. In fact, work is no longer viewed as work when one is fully engaged. No longer considered labor, work becomes a wellspring of joy and pleasure through intentional and purposeful effort to create or produce using one's unique natural talents and abilities.

An onlooker would be hard pressed to tell if a fully engaged individual is actually working or playing. That's because a fully engaged individual does not work. They are simply expressing who they are by what they do. They are demonstrating to the world their passion and purpose.

Engagement has the salient features of energy, involvement and efficacy, the exact opposites of exhaustion, cynicism and inefficacy. It describes a positive job-related state of mind characterized by:

- **Vigor** – reflects high energy, mental resilience, a willingness to invest effort in one's work and persistence in the face of difficulties. Keyword: **ENERGY**
- **Dedication** – a strong involvement in one's work with a sense of significance, enthusiasm, inspiration, pride, challenge and achievement. Keyword: **INVOLVEMENT**
- **Absorption** – happily engrossed and so concentrated in one's work that time passes quickly to a point where one has difficulty separating and detaching from work. Keyword: **EFFICACY**

Wow! Do you feel that way about your work? If you do, you are fully engaged. If not, well, maybe the time has come for some deep introspection and needed or necessary change. Why?

Engagement is a reflection of wellness.

Wellness is a dynamical state of self-awareness, healthy choices and a balanced life. *Shanafelt and colleagues noted:

*"Wellness goes beyond the absence of distress to include
being challenged, thriving, and achieving success
in various aspects of personal and professional life."*

A balanced life distills down your physical, emotional, intellectual, social and spiritual realms to crystallize you to your fullest potential so you become the fully elaborated version of YOU. Doesn't that sound awesome?

Even if you can not name exactly what you are looking for just now, if the words to describe it somehow seem too illusive, let me suggest it is just this — **a balanced life.**

"A balanced life brings us to the crossroads of our wants and needs, at the corner of passion and purpose."

*The asbtract of the Shanafelt article can be found at:
http://www.mayoclinicproceedings.org/article/S0025-6196(15)00716-8/abstract

The REIGNITE Framework
Taking the Necessary Steps to Alleviate Burnout

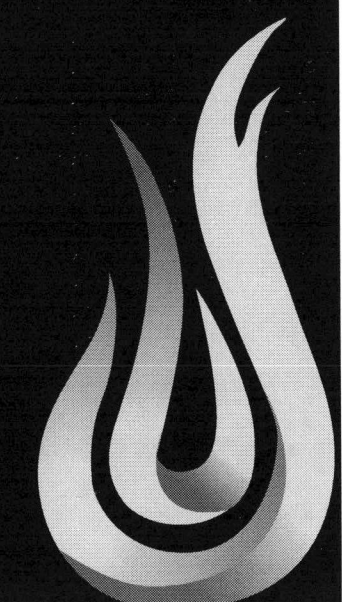

The **REIGNITE** framework is a stepwise process designed for mitigating, alleviating or eliminating the symptoms and causes of job-related burnout. Successfully completed, this process can transform an individual from burned out to ON FIRE with restoration of passion and a renewed sense of purpose.

The steps in this process are simple. They will serve as a guide. The degree to which each of the steps will help you will be based entirely on the effort you put into each of them. Be committed to getting the utmost from working each of these steps.

REIGNITE is your prescription for a balanced life.

As you go through each of the steps, be 100% willing to be transparent and authentic. This means becoming vulnerable. This will serve to ensure and secure the best possible outcome for you from this training.

Faithfully finish all of the steps you are asked to complete. It will be worth your time and effort. In the end, I am confident you will get far more out of completing the exercises in this workbook than you anticipate.

REIGNITE

Review – your current circumstances and the events that have led to them.

Envision – your brightest preferred future.

Introspection – taking inventory of your core values and honestly assessing the condition of all four of your life realms — mental, emotional, physical and spiritual.

Generate – ideas and action plans to transform your life.

Neutralize – all of the self-placed obstacles and barriers.

Implement – the plans you have made with a timetable of actionable steps with built-in accountability.

Transformation – acknowledging and documenting your progression from feeling burned out to a new freedom and a new happiness.

Engagement – celebrates a purpose-driven work life characterized by vigor, dedication and absorption while experiencing a more authentic and joyous life overall.

Let's go through each of these one by one.

The REIGNITE Workbook

Review

Review your current circumstances and the events that have led to them

How did you get to where you are right now? Looking back, what do you see as the major decisions, turning points or events that have lead you to where you are right now in your practice career?

_____
_____
_____
_____
_____

In life?

_____
_____
_____
_____
_____

Do you feel your practice career has negatively impacted your personal life or do you feel your personal life has negatively affected your career more? How so?

_____
_____
_____
_____
_____

Do you feel any of these circumstances are insurmountable? If so, which one(s)?

_____
_____
_____
_____

Is there one thing in particular over which you feel stuck?

_____
_____
_____
_____

The Hallmarks of Burnout

Which of the three hallmarks of JRB do you feel you have expressed?

Emotional Exhaustion – It is a feeling of being emotionally depleted to the point where you feel you can no longer give of yourself at an emotional or psychological level to your company or the people you serve. **KEYWORD: EXHAUSTION**

YES   or   NO

Depersonalization – The development of negative and cynical feelings leading to a callous and dehumanized perception of patients, clients or customers, which further leads to the view that they are somehow deserving of their problems and troubles. **KEYWORD: CYNICISM**

YES   or   NO

Lack of a Sense of Personal Accomplishment - You feel so little reward from what you do there is a tendency to evaluate yourself in negative terms, which leads to dissatisfaction and unhappiness in your work creating a lack of a sense of personal accomplishment. **KEYWORD: INEFFICACY**

YES   or   NO

Do your answers above square with your MBI results?

YES   or   NO

Were you surprised by the results of your MBI?

YES   or   NO

If yes, how so?

_____
_____
_____
_____

The Six Major Mismatches That Lead to JRB

Ninety percent of the time it is not the employee who burns themselves out, it is the work environment that burns out the employee. There are six major mismatches between the job and the employee, which lead to job-related burnout (JRB).

They are:

1. **Work Overload**
2. **Lack of Control**
3. **Insufficient Reward**
4. **Breakdown of Community**
5. **Absence of Fairness**
6. **Conflicting Values**

Many of the steps necessary to mitigate or alleviate the six major mismatches that cause provider burnout require changes at the business' organizational level. These are most easily accomplished in single provider practices or small group practices.

If you are an employee of a hospital or large provider group, changing the culture, management and organization of your employer may seem daunting or even impossible.

Nothing is impossible. It isn't about making your employer change. It is about leading them to a place where they want to change, a place where they feel that the proposed changes will benefit them. This can be easily demonstrated.

JRB causes increased costs and decreased profits by:

- Causing high rates of employee turnover
- Decreasing employee satisfaction
- Increasing employee absenteeism
- Increasing employee complaints
- Increasing customer complaints
- Decreasing the quality of products and services
- Creating hostile or toxic work environments
- Increasing lawsuits

**The direct costs of replacing just one physician can range from $150,000 to $1,000,000.
Direct and indirect costs can become staggering!**

The benefits of mitigating, alleviating and preventing JRB are modest in comparison. Here are just some of the benefits:

Eliminating or preventing job-related burnout will:
- Decrease employee turnover/Improve retention of needed talent
- Increase employee satisfaction/Decrease employee complaints
- Decrease employee absenteeism
- Improve customer satisfaction/Decrease customer complaints
- Increase the quality of products and services
- Eliminate work hostility and promote workplace harmony
- Decrease the threat of lawsuits

Bottom-Bottom Line: Decreased costs and increased profits!

Eliminating or preventing job-related burnout isn't just cost effective, it is income generating!

I ask you, what employer or CEO isn't interested in hearing that message?

Major Job Mismatches Self-Assessment

Which of the six major job-employee mismatches do you feel exist in your current work environment? Check all that apply. Then, for the ones you have checked, jot down one to three changes you would like to see occur, which would mitigate or alleviate them. Go further by making some proposals as to how those changes might be accomplished. Be as specific as you can be. Finally, make a commitment as to which of the proposals you will personally make attempts to see enacted in your workplace.

☐ **Work Overload** – Downsizing, budget cuts, layoffs, reorganization efforts all usually result in three things – more work intensity, more demands on time, more job complexity. In short, people are required to do ever more with less. This can leave individuals exhausted.

Needed Changes:

_____
_____

Change Proposals:

_____
_____

Commitment:

_____
_____

☐ **Lack of Control** – Organizations that become intolerant of creative problem solving in lieu of centralized control will squelch individual autonomy. This reduces an employee's capacity to set limits, exercise problem solving, select individualized approaches to work, allocate resources and set priorities. The overall effect is a loss of interest in the job and monumental frustration.

Needed Changes:

_____
_____

Change Proposals:

_____
_____

Commitment:

_____
_____

☐ **Insufficient Reward** – Market forces focusing on reducing costs have also reduced organizations' capacity to reward their employees in meaningful ways. People seek tangible rewards from meaningful work such as money, security, recognition, benefits, intrinsic satisfaction, etc. If these are lacking people naturally begin to wonder why they are working so hard. More work + less reward = dissatisfaction.

Needed Changes:
_____
_____

Change Proposals:
_____
_____

Commitment:
_____
_____

☐ **Breakdown of Community** – As organizations grow larger or grow too quickly, a breakdown in the character of the organization can result as short-term profit is chased at the expense of interpersonal relationships within the company. This will inevitably lead to greater conflicts among employees, a lack of mutual support, a lack of respect and a growing sense of isolation. Dr. Maslach states, "A sense of belonging disappears when people work separately instead of together."

Needed Changes:
_____
_____

Change Proposals:
_____
_____

Commitment:
_____
_____

☐ **Absence of Fairness** – Dr. Maslach perceives a workplace to be fair when three key elements are provided: *trust, openness, and respect. When all three are present, employees are valued and they will in turn feel valued and remain fully engaged (the opposite of burnout). When these elements are absent, burnout will be the direct end result..

Needed Changes:
_____
_____

Change Proposals:
_____
_____

Commitment:
_____
_____

☐ **Conflicting Values** – If organizations say they are dedicated to excellent service yet take actions that damage the quality of the services they provide, then conflict results. This can be extremely frustrating and demoralizing to the employee, especially if their internal moral compass or core values are being assailed. To achieve a quality product or service, a company's values must remain in alignment with those of the employees.

Needed Changes:
_____
_____

Change Proposals:
_____
_____

Commitment:
_____
_____

Do you feel these are present in your workplace?

TRUST   YES   or   NO

OPENNESS   YES   or   NO

RESPECT   YES   or   NO

Envision

Envision your brightest preferred future.

In this step you will envision your most desirable medical practice, practice venue, activities, relationships, living conditions and health status. In other words, I want you to envision what your life will look like one, three, or five years from now. It will be a picture of your preferred future.

You should know your preferred future is your dream and no one else's. Translating your life from where you are to your preferred future is your job. No one else will do this for you because they are concerned about their own lives and their own preferred futures.

It is time to cast aside your life of variations in sameness. It is time to choose for yourself a life without self-imposed limitations.

On the next few pages, you will begin to write down what your preferred future will look like. Not just your professional life but your family life as well. All four of your personal life realms will be included too.

Your entries won't just be ethereal someday hopes and dreams or pie in the sky aspirations. They will serve as concrete goals that you will work toward one step at a time, always asking yourself, "So, what's the next step?" until your goals are reached.

Remember, no holding back. No self-imposed limitations.

> **"If you can imagine it, you can achieve it. If you can dream it, you can become it."**
> ~ William Arthur Ward

"Your imagination can make you infinite."
~ A. C. Gaither

MY PREFERRED FUTURE

Describe what your ideal day would look like in the practice of medicine? How would you practice medicine? Full time? Part time? Solo? In a group? Physician owned or Corporate based? Would you stay where you are now?

_____
_____
_____
_____
_____

Where would you practice if you could practice anywhere your heart desired?

_____
_____

Where are you living? What kind of dwelling would you call home? What would your family life look like? What is your debt situation?

_____
_____
_____
_____
_____
_____

Are you working, playing or have you blended both so much an onlooker couldn't tell the difference? Are you a volunteer? A philanthropist? How will you be benefiting others? Who else will you serve and how?

_____
_____
_____
_____
_____

What emotional issues will you have finally dealt with as you enter your preferred future?

_____
_____

Describe your preferred health status. What healthy goals will you have achieved?

_____
_____

What outside interests, hobbies, activities are you enjoying in your future?
What will you be doing to expand your interests outside of medicine?

_____
_____
_____

What will your spiritual life look like? What changes have you made?

_____
_____
_____
_____

It is important to write these down completely on paper with attention to detail. To end up precisely where you wish to be, you must have some sense of where you are headed.

> **"If you do not change direction, you may end up where you are heading."**
> ~ Lao Tzu

I want you to be massively successful in whatever capacity you choose. The reason is simple. It will be much easier for you to give of yourself from a cup that is overflowing than from one that is never full or almost always empty. I want you to be able to serve and contribute to your patients, your family, your community, and to the world from a position of abundance rather than struggle from a position of scarcity. It begins first by caring for yourself, perhaps in ways you never have before.

Completing this step will produce a roadmap you will use to get you to your desired destination. This is a very important part of your **REIGNITE** journey.

Introspection

Introspection means taking inventory of your core values and honestly assessing the condition of all four of your life realms — mental, emotional, physical and spiritual.

If you have already completed a Core Values Inventory (CVI) then you already know your top five core values and your number one core value. If you have not yet completed the CVI, do so as soon as possible. Click HERE to download a free CVI that you can print out and complete at your earliest convenience.

The CVI is a process of self-discovery! Everyone has a set of core values that are integral to who they are or even to who they profess to be. Your core values may change throughout the different seasons of your life, but they are always with you. When you form an opinion, make decisions, or create judgments, you are either honoring or dishonoring our core values in the process.

If you are honoring your core values, you are more likely to be happy. If you are dishonoring your core values, you are more likely to be miserable. In violating your own core values, you will lead to burnout in your job, your personal life and on living.

To be a person of honor is to possess and display integrity in one's beliefs and actions. This is most easily accomplished through one's core values. This is why everyone should take a Core Values Inventory.

Knowing your core values will offer crystal clear insight as to who you are. This could be, should be, used as a guide when making both the large and small decisions affecting your life.

We all make choices. All of us will experience consequences as a result of our choosing. If we choose poorly for ourselves, the consequences are likely to be undesirable. Alternatively, choosing based on a true reflection of who we are will help to ensure more positive outcomes.

Core value guided decision making helps immensely when choosing a career, a particular job, a mate, friends, associations, even a home or a car. Deciding in this way, in favor of your own core values, promotes synergy between you and the life you choose to live. Synergy promotes harmony.

Everyone has been confronted at some point in their life with a situation, decision or request from someone that dishonors or goes against their inner compass or core values. Think back in your own life to whenever this has occurred. You probably said or thought something like, "I can't do that," or, "This is not me," or, "That's not who I am."

If you decided in your own favor, you were honoring the core values that were being challenged. Afterward, you probably felt good about your decision. If you went counter to what you were telling yourself at the time and made the decision to proceed against your better judgment, I am 100% certain you dishonored one or more of your core values.

Afterward, you probably felt bad about your decision. What was the ultimate outcome? How did decisions dishonoring your core values affect your life, positively or negatively? Conflicting values is one of the biggest of the six major mismatches between the job and the employee that create burnout.

When you look back at the decisions you have made that brought you to where you are now, were those decisions dishonoring your core values? If so, which decisions?

_____

_____

Deciding counter to our core values can lead to lying, cheating, stealing, burnout, bankruptcy, relationship problems and all of the attendant negative consequences. Laboring in a career or at a particular job that violates our core values will ultimately lead to burnout. Burnout reflects immense personal dissatisfaction and unhappiness.

Self-inflicted or job-related burnout is no state in which to live. It is impossible to live a life of purpose and passion burned out. The best way to avoid burnout is to celebrate and honor your own core values in everything you do and in every decision you make.

When you are getting ready to make a decision, large or small, consider first whether or not the decision or potential outcome is in line with your core values. Determining your top five core values, and your #1 main core value can be challenging but very enlightening and even enjoyable.

Your Mental Realm

Physicians are very good at feeding their mental realm, at least when it comes to medicine. How about outside of medicine? For many, not so much.

Medicine is a vast discipline, with an incomprehensibly large data base. No human could possibly know or learn all there is to know in medicine, or in a single branch of medicine for that matter. No human can keep up with all of the new information being published every single day. Yet, this does not prevent many physicians from trying. Thank goodness, anything you want or need to know in medicine is easily accessible now days.

Too many physicians' thirst for knowledge begins and ends within the discipline of medicine. It's a shame, really. There is so much more out there to know and enjoy about life. They have stopped being curious about the world. Too many miss the benefits of learning outside the discipline of medicine.

For instance, reading about bee and ant colonies can help you run and organize an office. Science fiction not only stimulates the imagination, it predicts the future. Books on art and philosophy give you insight into the human condition and why understanding behavior helps make your patients better, more so than a whole bag of pills. I once read a book on quantum electrodynamics, specifically about particle entanglement, which made me realize just how interconnected we are, with everything!

On top of all of that, these and other nonmedical topics are just plain interesting, if you're curious. Curiosity, exploring and learning should never stop with earning a medical degree, or be confined by it. If you aren't naturally curious, you can become curious with intention. It is a learned behavior.

Expand your knowledge base outside of medicine and you will expand your horizons. Here are the fundamental steps needed for addressing the obstacles, challenges, shortcomings, or barriers to **REIGNITE** your mind.

Stimulate and nourish your brain. These are one and the same.

First, unless you are watching something purely educational, turn off the television. Most of what is on TV is crap and will make you stupid. If you must watch something for mindless entertainment, keep it under an hour a day. But just remember, they don't call it mindless for nothing.

Second, I can't think of anything that will get your mind stimulated faster than reading great books! Pick an area of interest outside of medicine and read to find out what you don't know. You won't even know what you don't know, or what you need to know, until you start reading.

Dan Miller (48 Days to the Work You Love) suggests reading inspirational and uplifting books for at least thirty minutes each day. This is the best way I know to switch your brain to **REIGNITE** style thinking. This is something I do and wholeheartedly endorse.

Read nonmedical periodicals as well to stimulate your thinking. Foster a hobby. Read poetry and awesome quotes. Listen to a variety of music and podcasts that interest you. There is nothing of interest that I can't find on the Internet. I have made this bet countless times with friends. I always win. The world is at your fingertips through the world wide web.

Are you stimulating and feeding your mind daily? If not, why not? What are the barriers to learning that you perceive? Are they real or imagined? Answer here.

_____
_____
_____
_____

Do you read and explore for learning purposes outside the discipline of medicine on a regular basis?

YES   or   NO

If yes, what? _____

What do you wish you knew more about or had more time to learn outside the practice of medicine?

_____

Write down something you will commit to reading for learning outside of medicine on a regular basis.

Commitment: _____

Do you read for pure pleasure?   YES   or   NO

What was your last pleasure read and when? _____

If no, or more than one year ago, what will be your commitment for pleasure reading?

Commitment:
_____
_____
_____
_____
_____

Your Emotional Realm

This is the second-most ignored realm when it comes to physicians. Personal emotional health, and how to foster it, is just not something on which a lot of time is devoted during medical training. Yet, it is the realm that takes the heaviest toll when physicians and other health care providers burn out. The reason is simple. Mental anguish is often worse than physical pain.

Emotional exhaustion is one of the hallmarks of JRB. It is the first hallmark women usually feel and the second hallmark men feel. It occurs when the physician can no longer give of themselves to their patients on an emotional or psychological level. In essence, they become emotionally spent.

If the State of Happiness is a healthy mind, body and spirit, then the capital city would be Emotional Well-being. If your emotional well-being is suffering, chances are your mental, spiritual and physical realms are suffering too. How does one repair damaged emotional well-being? What kind of transformation does that take?

None of us are born emotionally damaged, ill or bankrupt, yet that will be how some of us end up. People can feel beaten up emotionally by others, by circumstance, by lack of success, by life and, of course, by burnout. Some people display tremendous hardiness and are resilient. They overcome emotional setbacks without long-lasting impact. They may even thrive after an emotional setback.

Others languish and may break down mentally, physically, and spiritually because of uninterrupted emotional turmoil. Seemingly unable to turn things around, they can become paralyzed by their emotional misery. When you are viewing everything through a corrupted and broken emotional lens, everything around you looks corrupted and broken too.

In the worst instances of emotional trauma, professional assistance may be necessary. If that sounds like you, seek professional help as quickly as possible. Know this — under the right circumstances and with proper care, everyone can heal.

But what is the difference between these two types of people — the ones who can seem to turn things around for themselves under the worst possible circumstances and the people who seemingly can't?

A twelve-year-long landmark study by a leading psychologist, Dr. Salvatore R. Maddi, found that those who thrived in spite of ruinous emotional stress possessed three key beliefs or traits that helped them weather adversity and turn it to their advantage.

It all came down to attitude: the **commitment attitude** that would lead them to act to be involved in ongoing events, the **control attitude** that would lead them to struggle to try and influence outcomes, and the **challenge attitude** that would lead them to view stressors, whether positive or negative, as new learning and growth opportunities. Dr. Maddi termed this **hardiness**. Others refer to it as resilience.

The operative word here is attitude. Is your attitude something that is handed to you by someone else, dictated by circumstance or something you are born with perhaps? No, like so much else in life, the attitude you have about anything and everything is a personal choice.

Good emotional health doesn't automatically fall onto you from the sky as you sit and contemplate all that is wrong with your life. **Emotional balance** is something that can be cultivated and developed. Like anything else in life that is worthwhile, it takes choosing differently for yourself, some effort, some practice, some patience and time.

Some might argue that this is easy to do for people who are successful. It is easy to be happy, hardy and more resilient when you are happy, right? Psychologist Dr. Sonja Lyubomirsky of the University of California, Riverside found that chronically happy people turn out to be more successful across many life domains than people that are less happy. Makes sense. The surprise was that their happiness was in large part a direct consequence of their positive emotions and attitudes rather than from their success.

The people he studied were happy before they were successful. They became more successful because they were happy. Here it is in a nutshell:

HAPPINESS = SUCCESS = HAPPINESS

It is time to state something clearly and unequivocally here. Everyone is entitled to their own emotions. Everyone should own their own emotions and be wholly responsible for them. It is then, and only then, that one is able to change them.

How do you make yourself happy? Well, I know how to do that for myself. I have no idea how to **make** you happy. That is your journey. I have a general sense of the what it might take to make happiness easier to obtain for most people who aren't happy.

Embrace, cling to, devour the positive aspects of living. Read poetry, uplifting books, inspirational stories. Improve yourself. Learn! Watch comedies. Laugh! Laugh some more. Laugh at yourself.

Are you hardy, resilient and happy? Or, emotionally unbalanced? Are you thriving or in need of emotional transformation?

Avoid negativity. Norman Vincent Peale once said, "Avoid like the plague those who fail to crystallize you to your full potential."

He is saying avoid negative people as you would a suppurative, plague-induced bubo draining pus. That's pretty emphatic. Surround yourself with positive people. Decide to become, at all costs, a positive person. It is but a choice after all.

A positive Transformation requires positive input. Negativity is anathema to positive change. No one would begin a race while tethered to the ground. Negative attitudes, beliefs, outlooks, forecasting, viewpoints, approaches and positions are just binders that keep us stuck. Whether they come from within or from outside ourselves makes no difference.

Make this pledge to yourself.

"I am going to become a more positive person by surrounding myself with positive and uplifting people, exploring and employing resources for positive thinking and behaviors while avoiding negativity like the plague."

Avoid negativity like the plague because it will poison the wellspring of your soul. This must begin within yourself first. This may take some getting used to if you have trained your brain to think or react negatively to any given situation.

Like any bad behavior that has been learned, negative thinking can be un-learned. It doesn't just happen by **trying** to think positively all of the time. It comes from **learning** to think positively and that means being proactive. Here are three steps to help you accomplish this.

1. Begin to read positive, uplifting, inspiring, challenging and affirming material. In whatever your area of interest, find great books and read them! Go to the websites of people you admire and search their reading list. Most will have one and you will begin to notice the wells from which they draw their experience,

strength and hope. Study their sources of inspiration.

If you live your life according to what is presented in the popular press, we are supposed to be afraid of something, in dire need of something, or eminently dying from something 24/7. Mainstream news is all about what is deficient, broken or missing. If there is an occasional feel good story, it is always used as a hook to get you to watch the gloom and doom forecast and reporting.

The Internet has greatly expanded out news source horizons. Look for blogs, websites and podcasts full of positive information that will help inspire, motivate and crystallize you to your full potential. Everything else is a distraction and a waste of your time.

2. Surround yourself with like-minded, purpose-driven, passionate people. Avoid negative individuals wherever possible or at least learn how to filter out their negativity. If someone offers you a negative sentiment or observation, don't waste energy disagreeing with it. Rather, try to rev up your positivity generator by countering their statement with a positive spin or comment.

3. Challenge and then change your attitude. Look for the positive in everything. Notice positive occurrences throughout your day and begin to comment on them out loud to others.

Try to go an entire day without making negative or derogatory statements. This does not mean that you are to stop giving or receiving constructive criticism. Honest constructive criticism is positive, good and helpful, not at all negative. You know the difference.

These steps will help you to regain control over any pessimism and cynicism that may be dogging you. Or, maybe your positivistic generator is just in need of a tune-up rather than an overhaul. Either way, taking ownership of this step of your transformation is sure to brighten your pathway to the future you wish to create for yourself.

How many hours per day do you watch television? _____

Commitment: _____ max.

How much time per day do you spend in meditation, prayer or quiet time? _____

Commitment: _____ (20 minutes minimum)

How many hours or minutes per day do you spend reading or listening to motivational or inspirational content? _____

Commitment: _____

Thinking about the people you hang out with most often, would you describe them as more (circle one) NEGATIVE   NEUTRAL   POSITIVE   ?

Are you a (or the) negative voice in a group setting?   YES   or   NO
If yes, how could you change this paradigm?
_____
_____

Do you have a colleague(s) who you confide in often?   YES   or   NO
If no, will you commit to finding someone with whom you trust? List three possibilities:
_____   _____   _____

How do you get your news? _____

Do you feel better or worse about the world after listening to the news?   BETTER   or   WORSE

If worse, what would be a solution for this?

_____

_____

Do you keep a journal? Would this be beneficial for you?

YES   or   NO   If yes, what will be your commitment for journaling?

Commitment: _____

Your Physical Real

As physically conditioned as they are, athletes know their game is mostly mental. As physically unconditioned physicians are as a group, how can we not know our game is as much physical as it is mental?

There is a part of TRANSFORMATION, which is often overlooked when most people begin to change their lives for the better and in profound ways — the physical realm. You will never be the best you can be, the best you can become, if your physical house isn't in order. Physicians are no different.

Completely transforming yourself and your life into the person you want to be, living the life you want to live, doing the kind of work you want to do is going to require some effort. Being physically fit will help you to accomplish the work that will be required to reach your goals. It's absolutely necessary and it will make your transformation a whole lot easier and much more enjoyable.

To be more mentally fit, you must become more physically fit. You might ask, what has one to do with the other? I have never seen a mentally fit person who felt as mentally sharp as they were capable of feeling if they felt poorly in their body.

Similarly, I have never seen a physically fit person who felt well in their body if they were suffering mentally. We all live inside our heads. What we "feel" is a summation of our emotional feelings and our physical feelings.

Furthermore, the sense of well-being that we all seek is a balance between all four realms — the mental, emotional, physical, and spiritual realms. Care for three and ignore one, and your life will be out of balance. The physical realm is the one most often ignored by doctors. Go figure. We recommend regular cardiovascular exercise to our patients but as a group we could do much better.

Trimming down, eating healthy, and regular exercise will make you feel great, like you can conquer the world! You will have more energy, more stamina, get sick less often and live longer. If you can't manage being totally fit, be as fit as you can be.

Regular heart-pumping exercise gives you a sense of calm and well-being that you can not get from a pill or a pep talk. Exercise boosts the immune system, clears the mind, lifts the spirits, and alleviates depression and anxiety. In short, it enhances your other three realms. Improving your physical health will improve all of them without any additional effort.

If you are going to transform, why not transform your physical status from unhealthy to healthy? It is never too late to start. Small changes add up and amplify over time.

If you have some health issues or are unsure of your health status, then be sure to consult with your own physician first to see what kind of diet and exercise program is best and safest for you. If you already enjoy the best health you can have for your age, you are one step ahead on your way to **REIGNITE**.

Do you have your own physician?   YES   or   NO

(You know what they say about doctors who treat themselves?)

If no, enter a date by which you will have obtained one.

Commitment: _____

Personal physician candidates: _____

If yes, do you follow your physician's instructions?   YES   or   NO

(There are two words for physicians who don't — noncompliant and hypocrite!)

Do you get regular check ups?   YES   or   NO

If no, enter a date by which you will have obtained a complete checkup.

Commitment: _____

Are you up to date on all of your health screen and health maintenance measures?   YES   or   NO   If no, enter a date by which you will be.

Commitment: _____

Do you do some type of regular cardiovascular exercise?   YES   or   NO

If yes, what?_____

(Claiming yard work, house work or a round of golf as cardiovascular exercise is like claiming you got useful information from a book you never read but just happened to walk past.)

If no, write down one form of cardiovascular exercise you will commit to doing regularly beginning ASAP (pending clearance from your doctor).

Commitment: _____

Do you hike, run or do water sports or something else outdoors regularly?   YES   or   NO   If yes, what? _____

In no, write down one outside activity you will commit to regularly.

Commitment: _____

Do you get adequate rest?   YES   or   NO

How many hours of sleep do you get each night on average? _____

Commitment: _____ (min. 7 ½ hours recommended)

Do you feel you need to lose weight?   YES   or   NO

If yes, what realistic amount will you commit to losing over the next one year with a proper diet and exercise program?

Commitment: _____

Have you been wanting to join a gym for exercise?   YES   or   NO

If yes, enter a date by which time you will have joined a gym.

Commitment: _____

Other ways you might improve your physical realm:

_____
_____
_____
_____
_____
_____
_____
_____

Your Spiritual Realm

No self-help assessment or effort can be complete unless you address the health of your spiritual self. If you are to **REIGNITE** your life, not just change it, then your spiritual realm is just as important as the other three realms. Maybe even more so. It is the deeper part of you.

The spirit encompasses your sense of who you are, why you are here and your place in the world. It represents your connectedness, or lack of connectedness, to other people, to nature and reality. Your spiritual health is reflected in your sense of purpose. Do you know why you are here? If not, are you still searching?

How is your spiritual health? Do you feel connected to humanity, a higher power, nature and the world around you? Do you have hope for the future, face each day with excitement, feel optimistic, a sense of peace, a sense of calm and serenity? If so, you are in excellent spiritual health.

Or, do you live in fear under a prevailing sense of dread, feel you walk alone in this world, prefer pessimism over optimism, feel hopeless or helpless, feel empty or apathetic and anxious for the future? Do you have unnamed or unreasonable fears? Do you feel you know who you are and have a sense of purpose? Or, are you somewhere in between these two extremes? If so, then your spiritual self may be damaged or suffering.

When I was an active alcoholic, my spiritual health was very poor. I felt dead inside. I felt it was impossible to change my circumstances, which gave me no hope for the future. I heard someone once describe how they felt when they hit their rocky bottom with drug addiction. He said he felt "perfectly broken." That is precisely how I felt, perfectly broken. Many of you may feel this way if you are instead "perfectly burned out."

There are many things that can enhance a damaged spirit or restore a broken one.

Be quiet and meditate every day. Concentrate on the things you do have rather than dwelling on what you don't have or feel you must have in order to be happy. Be grateful.

Get adequate rest! Play! Adults need to play just like children. Find ways to reconnect with your inner child. Color with crayons (especially outside the lines), draw, play with Play-Doh, run with scissors (okay, blunt ones), get in a tickle fight.

Sounds silly, I know. That's the point. Silly makes people laugh. Silly makes people smile. When you laugh and smile, you feel happy. It lifts your spirit.

You want to feel younger in five seconds or less? Get up out of your chair right now and skip! It will immediately make you smile or laugh. That is your inner child laughing. The spirit of a child is boundless and free. Your child-self is still inside you. It wants you to come out and play.

Practice mindfulness. If there is something you really enjoy, then really enjoy it. Slow down and savor everything worthy of your time and attention. Practice kindness, patience, the art of grace, empathy and compassion. Be decent and tolerant. Be honest. Tell the truth.

Study art. Start with what you like and then branch out. Take an art class. If you say that you aren't artistic and are of the opinion that artists are born, I will tell you that you are wrong. If artists are born, then there are just over seven billion of them on the planet and you are one of them. Take an art class and prove me wrong.

Listen to uplifting music. Again, start with what you like or are familiar with and branch out from there. If you can make music, make it and then make some more. Make music with others. Make music for others.

Connect with other people. Become part of a community. Well, except the Blah Blah Blah Nobody Loves Me Everybody Hates Me Community. That one is off limits. But, look around. There are so many different and interesting communities out there to which you can belong. Pick one that will capture your interest and keep you energized.

Connect with animals. Do you have a pet? Some of my most cherished memories are of my pets. There are powerful words and stories, which connect people and their pets. Pets can bring out the best in people. They will teach us valuable lessons if we let them. Do you have stories about a beloved pet?

Laugh. Laugh again. Laugh some more, especially at yourself. Go to a comedy club. Watch some of the old comedy shows that made you laugh when you were younger. You can find them all on the Internet these days. Carol Burnett, Harvey Korman, Tim Conway and Vicki Lawrence still crack me up. If I am feeling sad, all I have to do is pull up a YouTube clip and I am laughing out loud in less than a minute.

Give of yourself to others. Give your time. Volunteer. Help those less fortunate. Open your heart. Open your mind. In all things, try to be positive. Avoid negativity like it will kill you because it will if you let it. Share your most powerful words and stories with others.

Lastly, love yourself. You are not some pitiful, worthless creature to be loathed and despised, deserving of the worst the world has to offer. You are a luminous being, a child of the universe. My God, there is only one of you. There will never again be one of you. Laugh, love, live!

Do not deny yourself the wonders life in the world has to offer. You were born with God given talents and abilities that will allow you to improve any circumstance if you will but choose to do so. You may have forgotten this, but I haven't. The people who love you haven't.

How is your spiritual health?   POOR   GOOD   GREAT   AWESOME

Do you consider yourself a spiritual person? If yes, how so?

_____

If not, list three ways you could try to become more spiritual.

_____

_____

_____

Do you feel connected to the world and people in it?   YES   or   NO

If yes, GREAT! If no, list five things that you pledge to do, which will foster that sense of interconnectedness.

_____
_____
_____
_____

Do you take real vacations?   YES   or   NO

If no, I want you to plan a trip right now. I will go to _____

by _____ (within the next five months) for one full week minimum.

I pledge absolutely no working or CME while on vacation.

Signed: _____   Date: _____

Do you volunteer your time to a cause you support?   YES   or   NO

If not, is there one you could? _____

Do you go out into natural surroundings on a regular basis? If so, how?
_____

If not, list the kinds of outdoor activities that would interest you.
_____
_____

Do you go to museums?   YES   or   NO

If yes, what kind, where and when was the last time?
_____
_____

In not, if you were to pick one, where would it be and when?
_____

What would be your commitment for visiting a museum in the future?

Commitment: _____

Do you create art (a broad description)?   YES   or   NO

If so, what kind? _____

How often? _____

In not, what would you be willing to try and when?
_____
_____

Commitment: _____

Do you keep a journal? Would this be beneficial for your spiritual growth?

YES   or   NO   If yes, what will be your commitment for journaling?

Commitment: _____

Generate

Generate ideas and action plans to **TRANSFORM** your life.

As you know, nothing stays the same, ever. But most people want things to stay the same forever. Why? Where does that come from when it is completely outside of the human experience? I don't know.

Change is inevitable. Since it is inevitable, I believe it is better to try and choose your changes rather than have change choose you. It is a matter of planning, being proactive and intentional in our actions.

It is always nice to have options or choices. They are branch points on the decision tree of life that allow us to exercise some measure of control over our destiny. Sometimes options are numerous and we can pick our direction leisurely and without a lot of attendant anxiety.

Sometimes, our options are severely limited and we are forced to make hard choices. We have all been in the undesirable position of having to "choose the lesser of two evils." You may be there now. But, wasn't it a series of options and choices that put us in such predicaments in first place?

Ideally, it would be best to have more and better options most of the time with fewer instances where options are wholly constrained in scope with only frighteningly dreadful choices remaining. In this section, **you will begin to open up to the options that are available to you.**

The first step of **TRANSFORMING** your life is not a physical one. It is a mental step. It requires a change of your mind-set, a transformation in one's thinking. Win, lose, or draw, that is where the hardest battles are fought — in the mind.

There is also a difference between change and transformation. You can change your hair style, your clothes, your car, where you live, your job and your friends, but none of that will change you or who you are. When I talk about a transformation, I am talking about changes on the inside as well as on the outside.

Transformation isn't about becoming somebody different either. It is about becoming the more authentic version of you, living a life that is in concert with your core being, fully utilizing all of your unique natural talents and abilities. It is a metamorphosis.

Transformational change means fully elaborating your true self and acting accordingly. It all begins with accepting the notion "my life is not what I want it to be and I feel the need to change."

If you are ready, we will begin to generate ideas and action plans to **TRANSFORM** your life, which will take you from where you are into your preferred future.

In this step you will bring over action items that are the most important to you from the **MY PREFERRED FUTURE** section, pages 80-81. You will begin to list them in templates on the next several pages. For each category you will list each item under **Current Circumstance** and your preferred future outcome under **Desired Outcome**.

The really important action takes place in between, under Next Steps. Here you will begin to list what it will take to get you from where you are to where you desire to be. Getting from any point A to any point B is a progressive series of steps.

At this point, you do not have to precisely know every single step needed to get you to your desired outcome. You may inadvertently leave out a necessary step that is unknown to you at this time, or you might need to make adjustments to some of the steps as you go. Start with the most obvious and basic step first.

Then ask yourself, "What's the next step?" Then, "What's the next step?" and so on.

All of your focus and energy should be applied to writing out sequentially each needed step to reach your desired outcome. You can make adjustments as you go. Add new steps if needed. Never stop, though. Keep marching through them. Don't worry about filling in any start/stop dates just now. Those will be added later.

> "What a wonderful gift the universe has given us, the ability to transform."
> ~ A. C. Gaither

Action Item Template - EXAMPLE

Background: Dr. Clark Gaither is a fifty-four-year-old male family physician who completely burned out at his job after just seventeen years in private practice. He came to feel emotionally spent and exhausted. He grew cynical and felt he had nothing left to give to his patients who he began to resent much of the time. He felt as though nothing he did was making a difference anymore. He lived for the weekends and dreaded Mondays. Activities, hobbies and even the practice of medicine no longer interested him. He became irritable and moody at home. His family life began to suffer. He contemplated leaving the medical profession altogether until he participated in a workshop on job-related burnout. After acquiring the tools he needed to overcome burnout, he formulated a plan to alleviate his symptoms, corrected the underlying causes and recaptured the joy and pleasure of practicing medicine and balanced living.

Professional Life

Current Circumstance

Completely burned out at work, hate my job.   *Feb. 15, 2009*

Next Steps {
- *Cut down on work hours to 3 ten-hour days/week.*
- *Delegate nonmedical responsibilities at work.*
- *Resign from all board seats not passionate about.*
- *Get off extra, non-mandatory hospital committees.*
- *Identify several colleagues for support.*
- *Reduce call responsibilities.*
- *Volunteer more time in a free clinic.*
- *Restrict certain patients/procedures I don't enjoy.*
- *Restrict number of patients seen per hour.*

Desire Outcome

Enjoy medicine again, better attitude/outlook/energy.   *Mar. 15, 2009*

I was able to accomplish all of these goals within two weeks. The positive effects were immediate, profound and lasting!

Professional Life

Current Circumstance

_____   _____

Next Steps {
_____
_____
_____
_____
_____
_____
_____
_____
_____

Desire Outcome

_____   _____

_____
_____

Family Life

Current Circumstance

_____   _____

Next Steps {
_____
_____
_____
_____
_____
_____
_____
_____
_____

Desire Outcome

_____   _____

_____
_____

Mental Realm

Current Circumstance

_____   _____

Next Steps {
_____
_____
_____
_____
_____
_____
_____
_____

Desire Outcome

_____   _____

_____
_____

Emotional Realm

Current Circumstance

_____   _____

Next Steps {
_____
_____
_____
_____
_____
_____
_____
_____
_____

Desire Outcome

_____   _____

_____
_____

Physical Realm

Current Circumstance

_____   _____

Next Steps }
_____
_____
_____
_____
_____
_____
_____
_____
_____

Desire Outcome

_____   _____

_____
_____

Spiritual Realm

Current Circumstance

Next Steps $\Big\{$

Desire Outcome

Personal Debt

Current Circumstance

_____   _____

Next Steps {
_____
_____
_____
_____
_____
_____
_____

_____
_____

Desire Outcome

_____   _____

_____
_____

Social Arena

Current Circumstance

_____   _____

$\left.\begin{array}{l}\\\\\\\\\\\\\end{array}\right\}$

Next Steps
{
_____
_____
_____
_____
_____
_____

_____
_____
_____

Desire Outcome

_____   _____

_____
_____

The REIGNITE Workbook

_____

Current Circumstance

_____   _____

> _____
> _____
> _____
Next Steps
> _____
> _____
> _____
> _____
> _____

Desire Outcome

_____ _____

_____

_____

_____

Current Circumstance

_____   _____

Next Steps {
_____
_____
_____
_____
_____
_____
_____
_____
_____
}

Desire Outcome

_____   _____

_____
_____

The REIGNITE Workbook

_____

Current Circumstance

_____ _____

　　　　　　　　_____
　　　　　　　　_____
　　　　　　　　_____
Next Steps {　_____
　　　　　　　　_____
　　　　　　　　_____
　　　　　　　　_____
　　　　　　　　_____

Desire Outcome

_____ _____

_____

_____

_____

Current Circumstance

Next Steps $\Big\{$

Desire Outcome

The REIGNITE Workbook

_____

Current Circumstance

Next Steps $\Big\{$

Desire Outcome

_____

Current Circumstance

_____   _____

                _____
                _____
Next Steps { _____
                _____
                _____
                _____

                _____
                _____
                _____

Desire Outcome

_____   _____

_____
_____

Neutralize

Neutralize all of the self-placed obstacles and barriers.

"And the day came when the risk to remain tight in a bud was more painful than the risk it took to blossom."
~ Anaïs Nin

"My dear friend, clear your mind of can't."
~ Samuel Johnson

"One day, in continuous misery and feeling totally defeated, I had an epiphany. I came to realize, I had no place left to go, but everywhere. I had no one left to see, but everyone. I had nothing left to do, but everything."
~ A. C. Gaither, MD

No matter what new idea, notion, invention, innovation, product, service, business idea or change you might be considering, the first voice you will hear, the loudest voice you will hear, sometimes the only voice you will hear saying **STOP** or **NO** will be your own. Even now, this inner voice is saying things to you like "you can't," "you shouldn't," "it's impossible," "you're an imposter," "you're going to fail," "it's too late," or "you don't know what you're doing."

If you say "I can't," I will not believe you even though you will be right 100% of the time. My not believing that it is true will not make any difference, though, until you stop believing that it is true, at which point you will again be right 100% of the time. It is the only instance in your life when you will be 100% right either way. Your choice.

The words I can't or that's impossible form very finite statements. What would be, could be, should be begins and ends with those words. After those words, there is nothing left to add. They are declarations of cessation, of complete arrest and of conclusion. They are a barricade to further effort. The end.

Negative notions like "I can't" or "that's impossible" are powerful words. They hold people back and down of their own volition. They are dream stoppers and hope enders. The mere utterance of these words destroys initiative, stifles creativity and limits growth. They do not even have to be spoken in order to feel their full force. Just thinking these words is enough. How powerful is that?

For most people insisting on employing the "I can't" mentality, let's just get it right from the outset and translate this to what it actually means — "I won't." That might sound harsh but it's the truth. The truth only sounds harsh because it's the truth.

If you are full of discontent, unhappiness and discomfiture and are looking for a sign for when to begin to transform your life, your sign is discontent, unhappiness and discomfiture.

Do you often hear yourself say "I can't"? Was it last week? Yesterday? Perhaps today? Doesn't it shut you down cold? The only meaning to extract from "I can't" is "I am unable."

Saying "I can" means you are able to do something. This increases the potential that you will do something. Saying "I can" and taking action means no matter what the outcome, you have already won a different future for yourself.

What about the impossible? To say "I can imagine that's possible," would be the most likely opposing viewpoint. What I want to know is why some feel compelled to cry "impossible" before fully exploring what can be imagined to be possible?

The brain is an amazing organ. What it is unable to do, it can imagine doing. What can be imagined creates possibilities. Possibilities have a habit of turning into reality with time and effort. Which makes me wonder, exactly what can not be accomplished? I mean really?

Looking back, wouldn't you agree that much of what once seemed impossible is now not only possible but a reality. It's because someone dared to rethink the impossible.

If you have a goal in mind, is it the best one for you or have you compromised? Have you thought of other, better goals but rejected them because you felt they were too difficult or impossible? Why? Why do we limit ourselves so?

Look around. Those happy and successful people around you who made plans for brightening their own futures while brightening the futures of those around them harbored no thoughts of the impossible. In them, thoughts of the impossible are supplanted by "I have an idea," "Just imagine…" and "What if…"

Every happy and successful person, by whatever metric you wish to gauge these, has faced doubt, hardship, failure, struggle, ridicule, and fear. All of them. I submit none of them ever brought into their designs for happiness and success the words "I can't" or "That's impossible."

I can, I believe, I can imagine, and **that's possible** are all open-ended potential realities without limits. They are infinite in scope. They begin as words in someone's mind, mere thoughts, thoughts which will later become translated into action because new horizons are being envisioned, sweeping vistas sight unseen. Such thoughts will not be held back. They are too powerful.

It is time to choose for you a life without self-imposed limitations.
I want you to come to despise the orderly and unyielding flow of variations in sameness the words "I can't" and "that's impossible" seem to impose.

Make a list of five negative beliefs, objections or notions you have in your head that you feel are preventing you from taking the steps necessary to obtain your preferred future.

Negative Belief #1:
_____
_____

Negative Belief #2:
_____
_____

Negative Belief #3:
_____
_____

Negative Belief #4:
_____
_____

Negative Belief #5:
_____
_____

Now, I want you to make a list of possible solutions for each negative belief. If you have trouble getting started, try to think of what you would say to a friend who came to you for help with the same problem, someone you really wanted to help. If you get stuck on any one of them, ask for help from a positive, solution-oriented thinker. This could be a trusted friend, colleague, advisor, coach, personal physician, therapist or me.

Solutions to Negative Belief #1:
_____
_____

Solutions to Negative Belief #2:
_____
_____

Solutions to Negative Belief #3:
_____
_____

Solutions to Negative Belief #4:
_____
_____

Solutions to Negative Belief #5:
_____
_____

All negative beliefs regarding change should be approached in this manner. The big loud voice inside your head saying HELL NO will never go away, but it can be diminished.

"When it becomes more difficult to suffer than to change... you will change."
~ Robert Anthony

Implement

Implement the plans you have made with a timetable of actionable steps with built-in accountability.

Make a decision. Nothing will change for you until you decide it will change. Figuratively speaking, if you don't like the scenery, you can change the view. You must decide to decide things are going to be different.

Begin now. You are at the starting line of the rest of your life so start moving. You might not know exactly where the finish line is just yet, but at least you will be moving forward.

Help yourself first. Acknowledge your particular situation. Completely and honestly probe the depth and breadth of it. Know that you can be the agent of change in your own life. Stop waiting for outside forces to give you something, rescue you or provide for you. Help yourself first. Come to depend on yourself and your own actions for your own needs.

Ask for help if needed. I don't mean a friendly ear to bend or someone who will be content to offer words of encouragement. I mean people, agencies, facilities, providers, institutions, programs and groups that will offer assistance with your particular issues. This is not in disregard of the third step above. Asking for help if you honestly need help is helping yourself. You may need advice. You may need protection. You may need counseling. You may need treatment. You may need a coach. Ask for what you need.

Never turn back. I have seen people extract themselves from deplorable situations only to crawl right back to them in moments of weakness or self-doubt. Protect your weak spots. Develop strategies to protect yourself from the allure of old habits, codependency traps and situations that have harmed you. Your preferred future always lies ahead of you, never behind you.

Trust in change. You must come to realize that you are capable of more, that you can be different, create, learn, produce, build, and grow. We grow by how we change. We all have different natural talents and abilities that will compel us to change if we choose to use them. If you're not changing, you're not growing.

These steps are just the beginning to get you moving so you can begin to embrace the possibilities of change leading to a probability of success. They are intended to stop you from waiting for your future to just happen to you and to put you in control of it instead.

If you are ready to take charge of your future, I want you to go back to pages 108 - 121 and fill in some dates for each of the action items you have listed. Below is an example of one of the action templates.

Over to the right of **Current Circumstance** is a small blank space. Using your red pen, enter a firm date on which you will begin moving through your **Next Steps** for the action item listed. Over to the right of **Desired Outcome** there is another small blank space. Enter a reasonable target completion date by which time you will have completed the **Next Steps** and attained your **Desired Outcome**.

Professional Life
Current Circumstance

Next Steps {

Enter Begin By Date Here

Enter Goal Target Date Here

Desire Outcome

By entering a **Begin By** date, you are making a **COMMITMENT** to begin on that date. The completion date is an estimate. It's okay if you don't obtain the desired outcome by the exact date you have entered, but you must try your best if it is a reasonable time frame.

One way to ensure you are moving through your action items and steps is to have an accountability partner. This should be someone you trust who you will report to periodically or who will check on your progress. This should be someone who is positive, optimistic and motivated, someone who will both encourage and challenge you.

If you don't know anyone like this, then you need a new circle of influencers. If I'm coaching you, it would be me. Your accountability partner could also be a friend, colleague or advisor — someone other than a family member. This is too much of a responsibility to give someone who might have difficulty pressing you or being detached enough to be objective when necessary.

Make a list of possible accountability partners in order of preference right now and the exact date by which you will attempt to engage them for this important role. It's okay to have more than one accountability partner but no more than two. Use your red pen.

Potential Accountability Partners	Date I Will Attempt to Engage

It is a good idea to take the sheet(s) with your most important action items and post them where you can see them every day. Post them on your bathroom mirror, your refrigerator, the dashboard of your car, beside your computer at work (the places where you don't mind making them public).

Read over them every day. Keep moving through your Next Steps, always asking yourself, "What's the next step" that will move you toward your goal. Make any necessary adjustments as you go. Cross them off as you go so you can visibly see your progress.

First of all, you will be amazed just how much of your preferred future becomes reality when you write down your goals and begin to take clearly defined steps toward them. Second, you will be astonished at how quickly you begin to reach them.

Transformation

Transformation is acknowledging and documenting your progression from feeling burned out to a **new freedom** and a **new happiness.**

As I mentioned before, the first step of transformation is not a physical one. It is a mental step. It requires a change of one's mind-set, a transformation in one's thinking. Win, lose, or draw, it is where your hardest battles are fought — in the mind.

> "Transformation isn't about improving, it's about re-thinking."
> ~ Malcolm Gladwell

Although change and transformation are different sides of the same coin, they are as different as night is from day. You can change your hair style, your clothes, your car, where you live, your job and your friends, but none of that will change you, the real you.

Transformation isn't about becoming somebody different either. It is about becoming the more authentic version of you, living a life that is in complete alignment with your core being, fully utilizing all of your unique natural talents and abilities. It is a metamorphosis.

Transformation is not a one-off event. It is a mindset, a new way of living that is intentional and continuous.

Transformational change means fully elaborating your true self and acting accordingly. It is less about taking on a new persona and more about projecting your **true** persona to the world. You may need to **TRANSFORM** before you can **REIGNITE**.

If you have been crossing off your Next Steps and action items as you have completed them, you have seen the progress you have made, which is important. Monitoring your progress will boost confidence in your ability to adapt and change; rev up your ideas, innovation and creativity engines; open up a new universe of possibilities; and keep you on track as you march toward your preferred future.

There is another important benefit to **TRANSFORMATION** I haven't discussed up until now. Yet, it may be one of the most important reasons for you to transform, for anyone to transform for that matter.

This reason, should you decide to fulfill it, will become part of your legacy. I have no doubt it will help you answer the question, "Why am I here?" if you are curious to know. It is for this reason…

"Transformed people transform people."
~ Richard Rohr

I have always imagined I am here in this world, this big old universe, for a reason. You may have thought this too. Most people do.

I have come to feel I'm not here just to serve myself. I have long felt my purpose here is to help others on their journey in life, to pass along the best parts of myself and the best lessons I have learned, to help those who struggle and leave my corner of the world enhanced somehow by my being here. Ultimately, we serve ourselves in this way.

I don't have to ask because I already know — you also subscribe to this notion. Otherwise, you would not have chosen medicine as a career. I will tell you this, and it is undeniably true. You can never be your best at helping others and you can never live a life of passionate purpose if you are burned out.

"What is true passion without purpose? What is true purpose without passion? The combined fires of passion and purpose will never burn out, or burn you out, as long as they are conjoined."
~ A. C. Gaither

To live a life of purpose with passion, to be fully engaged demonstrating vigor, dedication and absorption while using all of your unique set of natural talents and abilities you must be **ON FIRE** for what you do. When you are, you will know firsthand exactly what I mean when I talk about a **new freedom** and a **new happiness.**

If you have **reviewed** your current circumstances, **envisioned** your preferred future, embraced **introspection**, **generated** ideas and action plans to transform your life, **neutralized** obstacles and barriers, **implemented** your plans with a timetable and accountability, then you are already undergoing a **transformation** and will on your way to **engagement**. You are ready to catch fire and **REIGNITE** if you haven't done so already.

Engagement

Engagement celebrates a purpose-driven work life characterized by **vigor**, **dedication** and **absorption** while experiencing a more authentic and joyous life overall.

Engagement is your goal. Not just for the immediate future, but for the rest of your life. Not just for your professional life, but for your personal and family life as well, in all four life realms — mental, emotional, physical and spiritual.

Engagement signifies a life in balance. A balanced life distills down your life realms and your unique set of natural talents and abilities to form a potent and powerful crystalline version of you, allowing you to reach your fullest potential.

To be engaged in all aspects of living is to become, as my publisher Jesse Krieger so eloquently describes, a fully elaborated version of you. This becomes the source of immense satisfaction as you live your life to the fullest.

We have identified the state opposite of burnout, which is **ENGAGEMENT**, characterized by **vigor**, **dedication** and **absorption**. The pathways to engagement can also be defined. There are six and they are the exact opposite of the six major mismatches which cause JRB.

According to burnout investigator and author [Christina Maslach](), the six pathways leading to **ENGAGEMENT** are:

1. **Sustainable workload**
2. **Feelings of choice and control**
3. **Recognition or reward**
4. **A sense of community**
5. **Fairness, respect, and justice**
6. **Meaningful and valued work**

Are any of these missing from your workplace? If so, circle in red the ones above that you feel are missing.

These can only be achieved if harmony is created between the employees and their employers in a way that leads to changes in the job environment as well as the workforce. Dr. Maslach has demonstrated very convincingly that burnout or engagement are foremost a function of the job situation and not the individual employee.

This is because individual employees can not for long carry the total burden of adjusting to fit their job or work environment. At some point, the job must begin to conform to the employee in a way that is conducive to engagement.

Focusing only on the employees who are burning out without a critical look at the work environment is counterproductive due to the economic law of diminishing returns.

This law states if one contribution (the employee's) in the production of a good or service (healthcare) is continuously increased and all other inputs are held fixed, a point will be reached at which additional contributions (work) by the employee will yield progressively smaller or even diminished results. This is where we are today in the medical profession.

When this occurs, employees will either become burned out or will be well on their way to burnout. To increase production at this point, one would have to change the entire work environment by making adjustments to every aspect of the production process. Some organizations are beginning to see this. Most are woefully behind.

This gets us back to the attributes that will define a healthy and engaged work force — a sustainable workload, feelings of individual choice and control, recognition of reward, a sense of community, fairness/respect/justice, and meaningful/valued work.

For large and highly entrenched groups or organizations, the process of building engagement may be difficult, but it is not impossible. I would say to the individual who loves their job but can not abide their current work environment that you can become the agent of change in your workplace.

As an initial step, I would suggest opening a dialogue with an administrator in your organization, whether it is a hospital or large provider group. They will rightly want to know what's in it for them. The approach that seems to be most useful is a discussion concerning resources — and by resources, I mean money.

The costs associated with JRB in toxic work environments can be devastatingly high. The benefits of fostering engagement in the workplace will add income to the bottom line and are therefore income generating.

Your discussion might also include a list of the major physician-job mismatches from pages 71-72 you feel are present in your current work environment, contributing to your burnout. These, along with the missing pathways to engagement from page 128, will give you a firm footing for a persuasive argument in favor of addressing JRB in your organization.

Pages 137-138 are from an Executive Summary I've prepared on JRB. This will be a useful tool for beginning a discussion with your employer on the advantages of eliminating JRB from your workplace and the benefits of nurturing workplace engagement. To download a PDF file of this document, click HERE.

Also, from my website at clarkgaither.com (Dr. Burnout) there is another document your organization's administrator might wish to download. It is entitled, "An Apple a Day Will Get the Doctor to Stay - 50 Low Cost or No Cost Ways to Keep Your Physicians Happy." It is a free download.

> **"You must be the change you wish to see in the world."**
> – Mahatma Gandhi

If you are burning out or completely burned out in your current work environment, it is incumbent on you to be the agent of your own change.

Either you must change or your work environment must change. Tough decisions and choices lie ahead.

If after hearing your concerns, your employer is unwilling to change and adjust the work environment, you may need to seek employment elsewhere in order to find a workplace more closely aligned with your core values and preferred future.

The alternative is to remain stuck in an environment where you can neither blossom nor thrive, a work environment you have come to despise. Moreover, it is a work environment that has called into question your thoughtful decision to enter your chosen profession for serving others — medicine.

I hope you will agree with me, working burned out is no way to live this one life.

What is your most favorite, inspiring, motivational quote? This would be a good place to write it down to serve as a reminder of your commitment to **REIGNITE**.

_____

_____

Job-Related Burnout
Executive Summary

The Problem: Job-related burnout causes increased costs and decreased profits by:

- Causing high rates of employee turnover*
- Decreasing employee satisfaction
- Increasing employee absenteeism
- Increasing employee complaints
- Increasing customer complaints
- Decreasing the quality of products and services
- Creating hostile or toxic work environments
- Increasing lawsuits

*The direct costs associated with replacing just one physician can range from $100,000.00 to over $1,000,000.00. Associated indirect costs will push this number even higher.

The Definition*: The three principle hallmarks of job-related burnout are:

1. **Emotional exhaustion** - It is a feeling of being emotionally depleted to the point where you feel you can no longer give of yourself at an emotional or psychological level to your company or the people you serve. KEYWORD: **Exhaustion**
2. **Depersonalization** - The development of negative and cynical feelings leading to a callous and dehumanized perception of patients, clients or customers, which further leads to the view that they are somehow deserving of their problems and troubles. KEYWORD: **Cynicism**
3. **Lack of a Sense of Personal Accomplishment** - You feel so little reward from what you do there is a tendency to evaluate yourself in negative terms, which leads to dissat-

isfaction and unhappiness in your work creating a lack of a sense of personal accomplishment. KEYWORD: **Ineffi-cacy**

*Note: Men and women go through these differently.

The Causes: 90% of the time it is not the employee who burns themselves out, it is the work environment that burns out the employee. There are six major mismatches between the job and the employee, which lead to job-related burnout:

1. Work Overload
2. Lack of Control
3. Insufficient Reward
4. Breakdown of Community
5. Absence of Fairness
6. Conflicting Values

The Cure: Programs and training designed to detect and mitigate any job-employee mismatches causing burnout or to prevent job-related burnout in the first place through:

- Instruction
- Workshops
- Measuring
- Programs to eliminate, mitigate and prevent employee burnout
- Monitoring
- Ongoing management

The Reward: Eliminating or preventing job-related burnout will:

- Decrease employee turnover/Improve retention of needed talent
- Increase employee satisfaction/Decrease employee com-

plaints
- Decrease employee absenteeism
- Improve customer satisfaction/Decrease customer complaints
- Increase the quality of products and services
- Eliminate work hostility and promote workplace harmony
- Decrease the threat of lawsuits

Bottom-Bottom Line: Decreased costs and increased profits

Eliminating or preventing job-related burnout isn't just cost effective, it is income generating!

Closing Thoughts

If you have been serious, intentional and steadfast in your approach to the steps outlined in this workbook, you are now better positioned to attain engagement exemplified by a life that is both resilient and balanced.

Remain flexible as you journey on. The unexpected will occur. Priorities will shift. Your mind will change about some things as you go because you will change as you move through different seasons of your life.

You will live longer if you keep setting goals. You should make 1, 3, 5, 10, 15, 25-year plans and beyond. Write your goals down using the action templates provided in this workbook (pages 101-103). Post them around and look at them often. Make a habit to keep asking yourself, "What's the next step? What's the next step?" as you move toward each goal.

Revise your goals periodically. Remove the ones you have obtained and make sure those that remain are still in alignment with your core values and the preferred future you desire. You will be amazed at your progress.

Just remember, whatever you choose will be. Mind-set is everything and you are in charge of you.

Let this be the beginning of a process, not the end of one.

Keep your eye on the prize — your preferred future.

With PASSION and PURPOSE,

REIGNITE

Products and Services

My website is at clarkgaither.com. I regularly post content there on all facets of job-related burnout. Only the most current, up-to-date information is presented.

Numerous helpful downloads are available for individual physicians and for hospital or group administrators who are interested in this topic, and they are all FREE.

Other products and services are also available for purchase. If you are interested in any of these products and services, please contact me directly. All of my contact information is listed below.

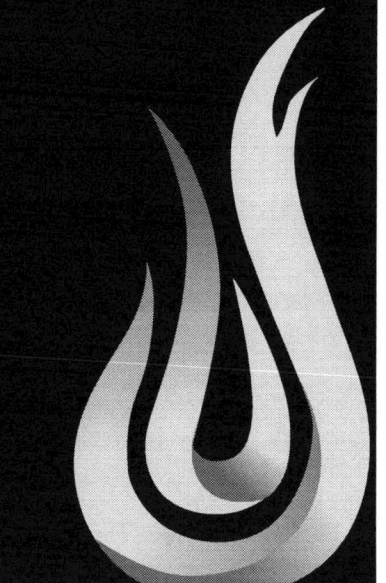

Clark Gaither, MD, FAAFP
(a.k.a. Dr. Burnout)

- Individual Coaching

- Group Coaching
- Workshops
- Corporate Training/Consulting
- Keynote Speaker

Contact Information
Website: clarkgaither.com
LinkedIn: https://www.linkedin.com/in/clarkgaither
Facebook: https://www.facebook.com/drburnout
Twitter: @clarkgaither

Bio

Hello.

My name is Dr. Clark Gaither (a.k.a. Dr. Burnout) and I am a board certified family physician. A graduate of East Carolina School of Medicine, I have been in private practice in Goldsboro, NC, for the past twenty-four years.

Throughout my practice career I have given over a thousand talks on various topics including hypertension, cholesterol disorders, addiction and recovery issues, smoking cessation, various pharmaceutical therapeutic agents, and work-life balance.

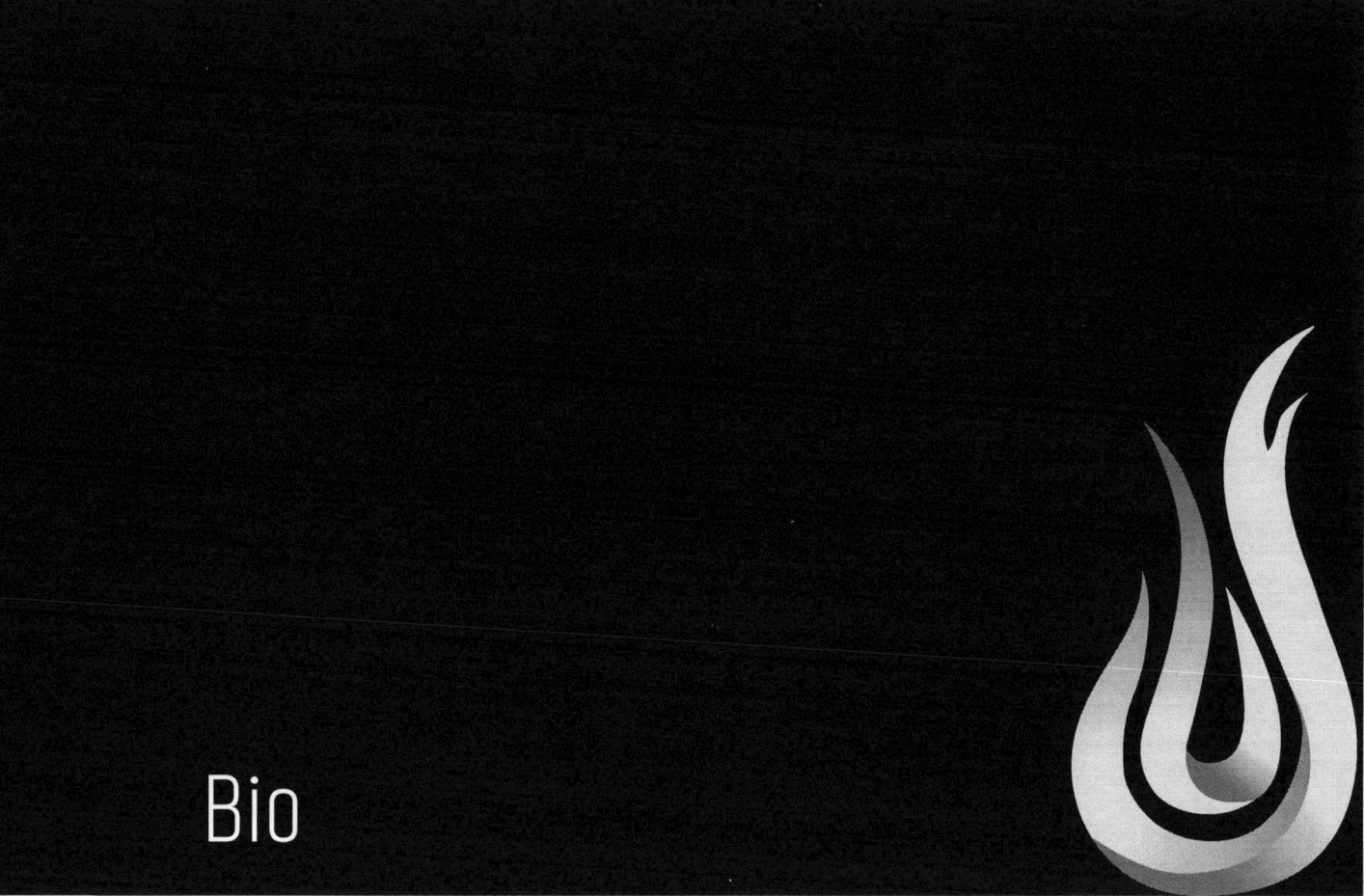

Clark Gaither, MD, FAAFP
(a.k.a. Dr. Burnout)

I am an author, speaker, blogger, personal life coach, consultant and artist. I have authored two books, *POWERFUL WORDS and The Graduate's Handbook — Your No Nonsense Guide for What Comes Next.* My third book, *REIGNITE — From Burned Out to ON FIRE,* will be out later this year.

For the last seven years, I have devoted myself to helping physicians, and other professionals, recover from the savages of job-related burnout. Having burned out and recovered from burnout myself, I can speak first hand and with authority on this topic. I am keenly aware of the devastation this condition can cause if not properly mitigated, treated and prevented.

If you were to ask me what I have been most proud of during my practice career, besides my work with burned out physicians, I would say it is this. In 2001, I created Wayne County's first free healthcare clinic. Endowment funds were obtained to put into service a mobile medical unit that serves our citizens at nineteen different locations each month. I volunteer on the mobile unit and continue to serve as medical director. Because of increasing demand, two free-standing satellite clinics were also created.

The patients we see in the clinics do not have healthcare benefits and do not qualify for benefits. With physician assistants and volunteers — physicians, nurses, students, hospital volunteers, members of the community — the services we provide include acute care and ongoing chronic disease management. With an annual operations budget of over $900,000, all of the care provided to our patients is free. Their labs are free and many of their medications are free. The clinics see 1,000 plus patients per month combined. To date, we have logged over 100,000 patient visits, serving 20,000 plus individual patients while providing over $2,000,000 in free pharmaceuticals. It is the second busiest free clinic in North Carolina.

In 2002, I was honored as Family Physician of the Year by the NC Academy of Family Physicians and nominated for the AAFP's Family Physician of the Year. In 2010, I became a Fellow of the

American Academy of Family Physicians.

There are many other interests that enrich my life immensely, and I also consider them just plain fun. I love to run, hike and travel. You can find me underwater scuba diving at many blue water destinations or under clear night skies at the eyepiece of my telescope enjoying amateur astronomy. I do wood and metal art and I have been making furniture since I was fifteen years old. I collect rocks, minerals, and meteorites. Writing has become one of my most favorite pastimes.

I currently live with my trusty and most excellent companion, Eli. I would be remiss, and Eli would be disappointed, if I didn't include his picture here.

Made in the USA
Lexington, KY
22 October 2016